LASIK

COMPLICATIONS

PREVENTION AND MANAGEMENT

SECOND EDITION

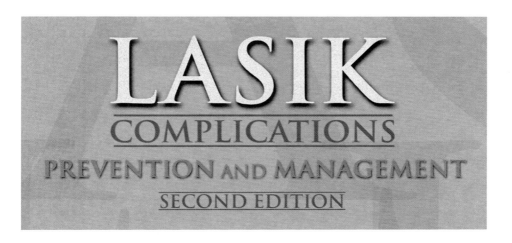

LASIK COMPLICATIONS
PREVENTION AND MANAGEMENT
SECOND EDITION

Howard V. Gimbel, MD, MPH, Diplomate ABO, FRCSC
Professor and Chair, Dept. of Ophthalmology
Loma Linda University, Loma Linda, California

Gimbel Eye Centre
Calgary, Alberta, Canada

Ellen E. Anderson Penno, MD, MS, Diplomate ABO, FRCSC
Research Advisor and Associate Director of Research Publications, Staff Surgeon
Gimbel Eye Centre
Calgary, Alberta, Canada

ASSOCIATE EDITORS
N. Timothy Peters, MD
Refractive Surgery Fellow, Gimbel Eye Centre
Calgary, Alberta, Canada

Nader G. Iskander, MD, Diplomate ABO
Refractive Surgery Fellow, Gimbel Eye Centre
Calgary, Alberta, Canada

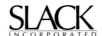

SLACK
INCORPORATED

an innovative information, education, and management company

6900 Grove Road • Thorofare, NJ 08086

Publisher: John H. Bond
Editorial Director: Amy E. Drummond
Design Editor: Lauren Biddle Plummer

The procedures and practices described in this book should be implemented in a manner consistent with the professional standards set for the circumstances that apply in each specific situation. Every effort has been made to confirm the accuracy of the information presented and to correctly relate generally accepted practices. The author, editor, and publisher cannot accept responsibility for errors or exclusions or for the outcome of the application of the material presented herein. There is no expressed or implied warranty of this book or information imparted by it.

Care has been taken to ensure that drug selection and dosages are in accordance with currently accepted/recommended practice. Due to continuing research, changes in government policy and regulations, and various effects of drug reactions and interactions, it is recommended that the reader review all materials and literature provided for each drug, especially those that are new or not frequently used.

Any review or mention of specific companies or products is not intended as an endorsement by the author or the publisher.

Gimbel, Howard V.
        LASIK complications: prevention and management/Howard V. Gimbel, Ellen E. Anderson Penno.-- 2nd ed.
                p. ; cm.
        Includes bibliographical references and index.
        ISBN 1-55642-473-6 (alk. paper)
        1. LASIK (Eye surgery) Complications. I. Penno, Ellen E. Anderson. II. Title.
        [DNLM: 1. Keratomileusis, Laser In Situ--adverse effects. 2. Postoperative Complications--prevention and control. 3. Refractive Errors--surgery. WW 220 G491L 2000]
        RE336 .G54 2000
        617.7'19059-- dc21   00-041933

Printed in Colombia.

Published by: SLACK Incorporated
                       6900 Grove Road
                       Thorofare, NJ 08086 USA
                       Telephone: 856-848-1000
                       Fax: 856-853-5991
                       www.slackbooks.com

Contact SLACK Incorporated for more information about other books in this field or about the availability of our books from distributors outside the United States.

Authorization to photocopy items for internal or personal use, or the internal or personal use of specific clients, is granted by SLACK Incorporated, provided that the appropriate fee is paid directly to Copyright Clearance Center, 222 Rosewood Drive, Danvers, MA 01923 USA, 978-750-8400. Prior to photocopying items for educational classroom use, please contact the CCC at the address above. Please reference Account Number 9106324 for SLACK Incorporated's Professional Book Division.

For further information on CCC, check CCC Online at the following address: http://www.copyright.com.

Last digit is print number: 10   9   8   7   6   5   4   3   2   1

Dedication

To our spouses and families,
for their love and support.

Contents

Acknowledgments

This project could not have been completed without the tireless assistance of Mae Jensen, Fern Sinclair, and the rest of the research staff.

About the Authors

Howard V. Gimbel, MD, MPH, Diplomate ABO, FRCSC

Howard Gimbel is the Founder, Medical Director, and Senior Surgeon of the Gimbel Eye Centre in Calgary, Canada. Dr. Gimbel received his doctorate in medicine and a masters in public health from Loma Linda University in California. He completed his internship and ophthalmology residency at the White Memorial Medical Center in Los Angeles. In 1964, Dr. Gimbel began practicing as an eye specialist in Calgary. Dr. Gimbel has academic appointments at University of Calgary, University of California-San Francisco, and is Professor and Chairman of the Department of Ophthalmology at Loma Linda University.

Gimbel Eye Centre-Calgary was the first center in Canada to perform excimer laser photorefractive keratectomy (1990). Since that time, Gimbel Eye Centre surgeons have performed over 25,000 laser vision correction procedures. Dr. Gimbel has personally performed over 10,000 vision correction procedures. Dr. Gimbel is also Medical Director of Gimbel Vision International, a publicly traded Canadian company which owns and operates vision correction centers with affiliates worldwide.

Ellen E. Anderson Penno, MD, MS, Diplomate ABO, FRCSC

Ellen Penno joined Gimbel Eye Centre-Calgary after completing a 1-year refractive surgery fellowship at Gimbel Eye Centre. Building upon an extensive research background at the Mayo Clinic in Rochester, Minnesota in 1998, Dr. Penno was appointed the Corporate Director of Research for Gimbel Eye Centres in Canada.

Dr. Penno brings a valuable mix of education and experience to ophthalmology. Fulfilling a lifelong ambition, Dr. Penno graduated from the University of Minnesota in 1992 with a combined medical degree and master's degree in clinical laboratory science, and in 1996 completed a 3-year residency at the internationally recognized Mayo Clinic. Following residency, Dr. Penno spent 1 year practicing as a general ophthalmologist in Sedona, Ariz. In private practice in Arizona, she performed refractive surgery and clear corneal cataract surgery. Dr. Penno has coauthored numerous publications and book chapters relative to refractive surgery, including *Refractive Surgery: A Manual of Principles and Practice.*

N. Timothy Peters, MD

Tim Peters completed a fellowship in refractive surgery at the Gimbel Eye Centre in 2000. Originally from California, Dr. Peters has traveled the country during his training. He graduated in 1991 from the University of California at Davis with honors and a degree in human physiology. Dr. Peters received his doctorate in medicine from Baylor College of Medicine in Houston in 1995. He completed his internship at the University of Hawaii in 1996, and then completed a residency program in ophthalmology at the University of California at Irvine in 1999.

Dr. Peters adds his experience in surgical and research activities to the team. He has authored numerous publications on ophthalmology and given lectures on refractive surgery at major international ophthalmology meetings. Dr Peters is currently the director of refractive and anterior segment surgery at Nationwide Vision in Phoenix, Arizona.

Nader G. Iskander, MD, Diplomate ABO

Nader Iskander completed his fellowship training at the Gimbel Eye Centre. Originally from Egypt, Dr. Iskander obtained his General Certificate of Education from the University of London England in 1983. Dr. Iskander received his doctorate in medicine with honors from Alexandria University Medical School in 1990. He trained in internal medicine at the Cleveland Clinic between 1993 and 1995. He then completed his residency training in ophthalmology at the Kresge Eye Institute at Wayne State University in Detroit, Michigan in 1998. He joined the Department of Ophthalmology at Wayne State University as an Assistant Professor in 1998. Dr. Iskander is currently the associate director of the ophthalmology residency program at Wayne State University. He is also a refractive and anterior segment surgeon at the Kresge Eye Institute in Detroit, Michigan.

Dr. Iskander brings his global perspective to this team of refractive surgeons. He has written several publications on refractive surgery and lectured at different major international ophthalmology meetings.

Contributing Authors

Ashley Behrens, MD   Irvine, California
Dennis A. Braun, OD   Saskatoon, SK
Lawrence Chao, MD   Irvine, California
Roy S. Chuck, MD, PhD   Irvine, California
Daniel S. Durrie, MD   Kansas City, Missouri
Angela Q. King, MD   Winter Park, Florida
Damien C. Macaluso, MD   Portland, Oregon
Scott M. MacRae, MD   Portland, Oregon
Jaime R. Martiz, MD   Houston, Texas
Marguerite B. McDonald, MD   New Orleans, Louisiana
Lee H. Novick, MD   Irvine, California
Trent L. VandeGarde, MD   Kansas City, Missouri

Foreword

The history of LASIK (laser in situ keratomileusis) is the story of the evolution of lamellar keratoplasty, starting with Dr. Jose Barraquer in 1949. In that year, the very first studies of lamellar keratoplasty were performed in Bogota, Colombia. These studies formed the basis of today's LASIK procedure.

In 1958, Dr. Barraquer experimented with his flap technique and created positive and negative lenticules after freezing the excised lamellar stromal tissue. He also experimented with a planar stromal cut using a prototype of the microkeratome. This was also the first year in which corneal lenticules were implanted intrasomally for refractive correction.

In 1962, the microkeratome had evolved into a more sophisticated device with a 26-degree cutting angle, a pneumatic ring and track, and an applanation tonometer. The first intraoperative keratometer was introduced to evaluate the refractive change. In this year, the first cryolathe was invented and its algorithms defined. This year also marked the first intraoperative use of a computer in refractive surgery.

In the following years, Dr. Barraquer replaced his electronic calculator with a computerized system and designed a more innovative computerized cryolathe.

In 1977, Dr. Richard Troutman introduced keratomileusis to the United States when he brought a Barraquer cryolathe to the Manhattan Eye, Ear, and Throat Hospital in New York City. His former cornea fellow, Dr. Casmir Swinger, worked with Dr. Barraquer and Dr. Jorge Krumeich to perfect the BKS 1000 system for nonfreeze keratomileusis in situ.

In 1983, Stephen Trokel published his classic paper in the *American Journal of Ophthalmology* indicating that, based on his laboratory experiments with cadaver animal eyes, the excimer laser could be harnessed for corneal applications. In early 1984, while working with Trokel and Charles Munnerlyn, I began the first PRK experiments on animals. Shortly thereafter, I had the honor of performing the first PRK in the world on both blind eyes and sighted eyes (1987 and 1988).

In 1989, Dr. Lucio Buratto used photoablation on the exposed stromal bed of fully functional human eyes. After the creation of a free corneal flap, he experimented with laser application to the underside of the flap as well.

In 1990 and 1991, Dr. Ioannis Pallikaris of Crete developed LASIK as we know it today, using a hinged flap technique. Shortly thereafter, Drs. Avalos and Gumaraes developed the sutureless technique for LASIK.

In 1991, Dr. Stephen Brint performed the first LASIK procedure in the United States. Drs. Stephen Slade, Charles Casebeer, and Luis Ruiz refined LASIK and began teaching modern lamellar refractive surgery in the United States and abroad through organized practical courses.

In 1996, Dr. Lucio Buratto initiated the down-up LASIK technique, otherwise known as the superior hinge technique or top hinge LASIK.

By mid-1998, LASIK achieved worldwide acceptance as a means of correcting a wide range of refractive errors with good predictability, virtually no postoperative pain, and rapid return of visual acuity.

The first edition of this book was a huge success, for several reasons. First, this text is encyclopedic in its approach to LASIK complications. Second, as an introduction to LASIK, it is straightforward and easy to understand. Third, as a complete reference source for experienced LASIK surgeons seeking help with rare complications, it is unsurpassed.

LASIK is a science and an art, and while there are those with a natural gift for advanced refractive surgery, the skills are indeed transferable if presented properly to the motivated student. Teaching microsurgery is a special talent of Dr. Gimbel's, a fact that is appreciated by his many grateful students throughout the world. Thousands have visited the Gimbel Eye Centre in Calgary to watch him implement his principles in the operating room, as well as the examination lane.

LASIK surgeons at all stages of development have remarked upon the detailed case presentations of intraoperative and postoperative complications and their management, which are included in this textbook. High quality color reproductions of slit lamp photographs and videokeratographs greatly enhance these narratives. I know that his readers will enjoy and treasure this second edition of Dr. Gimbel and Dr. Penno's text, and keep it within arm's reach in their offices.

Marguerite McDonald, MD, FACS
Clinical Professor of Ophthalmology at Tulane University School of Medicine
Director, Southern Vision Institute
New Orleans, Louisiana

Preface

The second edition of this book on LASIK complications is prompted by the enthusiastic response to the first edition, as well as the desire to keep the book current as new methods and instrumentation evolve to help prevent and manage LASIK complications.

More and more refractive surgeons are benefitting from anterior segment and corneal fellowships that include LASIK technique training as part of the curriculum. In addition, refractive surgery fellowships are becoming available to provide indepth training in LASIK techniques. However, LASIK is a surgical technique that many surgeons still have to make the transition to without the benefit of such indepth training.

This book is a description, in as much detail as possible, of the subtleties and nuances of LASIK techniques and hopefully covers more information than is available in a short LASIK course. The focus of this second edition is still to warn of complications and review procedures and techniques, as well as how to manage the complications of LASIK surgery.

We welcome criticisms and suggestions of alternative techniques and additional experiences. The more we share, the more we learn, and the better the potential outcome for each of our patients.

Section I

LASIK Complications: Prevention and Management

1

The Changing Role of LASIK: Combined Sequential Refractive Surgery

Introduction

As the new millennium begins, refractive surgeons must become proficient in a wide range of corneal techniques including corneal ablative, lamellar, incisional, and thermokeratoplasty. Intraocular methods such as refractive lensectomy and phakic intraocular lens (IOL) implantation are also undergoing rapid refinement and are becoming the modality of choice for the correction of refractive errors in select patients. In spite of the wide array of choices, laser in situ keratomileusis (LASIK) remains the most popular choice of patients and surgeons as a primary technique. At our five centers across Canada, 81% to 91% of the procedures are LASIK, 2% to 3% photorefractive keratectomy (PRK), 5% to 13% refractive lensectomy, 0% to 1% intrastromal corneal ring segment implantation, and 0% to 2% phakic IOL implantation (Table 1-1).[1] LASIK cases account for up to 98% of total cases at our centers where PRK and LASIK are the only two options available.[1]

Refractive surgery patients and patients presenting for cataract surgery have increasingly higher expectations. Over the past two decades we have learned to combine intraocular and corneal surgery in the form of IOL implantation and astigmatic keratotomy (AK), as well as IOL implantation following previous

Table 1-1

Estimates of Refractive Surgeries Performed

Procedure	Percent
LASIK	81 to 91
PRK	2 to 3
Refractive lensectomy	5 to 13
Intrastromal corneal ring segments	0 to 1
Phakic IOL	0 to 2

These estimates are combined from five centers. At our centers, which offer solely excimer laser options, LASIK cases account for up to 98% of the total.

Table 1-2

Refractive Procedures

Procedure introduced at Gimbel Eye Centre

RK (radial keratotomy)	1983
AK (astigmatic keratotomy)	1983
PRK (photorefractive keratectomy)	1990
LASIK (laser in situ keratomileusis)	1995
ICL (implantable contact lens)	1997

Table 1-3

Combined Refractive Procedures

Corneal - IOL	*Corneal - Corneal*
AK during cataract	PRK after RK/AK
AK during lensectomy	PRK after LASIK
AK after lensectomy	LASIK after PRK
Cataract after RK	LASIK after AK
Cataract after PRK	AK after LASIK
Cataract after LASIK	
Lensectomy after RK	
Lensectomy after PRK	
Lensectomy after LASIK	
ICL after AK	
LASIK after ICL	
AK after ICL	

corneal refractive surgery (Table 1-2).[1-4] Increasingly we have used LASIK following phakic IOL and combined corneal-corneal refractive surgical procedures to optimize outcomes (Table 1-3).[5] Specific examples of mixed enhancements and retreatments are presented in Chapter 8 and in Section 2: Patient Examples.

Planned combined sequential refractive surgery will become more commonplace as surgeons gain experience in newer techniques and learn which combina-

Table 1-4
Time Line of Refractive Surgery

1980	PERK STUDIES
1983	Trokel and Srinivasan: Excimer laser demonstrated on bovine corneal tissue
1985	Seiler: First photorefractive keratectomy on a blind human eye
1986-present	Fechner, Worst, Baïkoff, Fyodorov: Design modifications of anterior and posterior chamber phakic IOL implants
1986	Modern anterior and posterior chamber ICLs
1987	Seiler: First PRK on a sighted human eye (slated for exenteration 11 days after PRK)
1988	McDonald: First PRK on a normal sighted human eye
1989	Pallikaris: Laser ablation under flap, "LASIK" coined
1990	Seiler, et al: Ho:YAG laser thermokeratoplasty correction of hyperopia up to +5 D
1991	First intrastromal corneal ring implanted in sighted eye (Brazil)
1991	Ruiz: Automated corneal shaper
1992	Buratto: Excimer under a cap
1995	Alternative intrastromal corneal ring design (ISCRS) introduced into clinical trials
1995-1996	Development of noncontact laser thermokeratoplasty
1999	Seiler: First customized corneal ablation in the world

(Reprinted with permission from Gimbel HV, Anderson Penno EE. LASIK Complications: Prevention and Management. Thorofare, NJ: SLACK Incorporated, 1999.)

tions provide the best possible visual result. For example, as Dr. Roberto Zaldivar suggests, creation of a LASIK flap followed by implantation of a phakic IOL enables the surgeon to easily adjust the postoperative result by simply lifting the flap and performing the desired laser ablation.[6] Zaldivar has termed this approach "bioptics."[6] Güell uses "adjustable refractive surgery."[7] This approach may be necessary to safely treat extreme myopia in younger patients who are not lensectomy candidates. However, as the array of applications widens, understanding the specific complications and appropriate techniques for avoiding those complications will become more complex. Expertise in each technique will provide a solid basis upon which to practice combined sequential refractive surgery.

BACKGROUND

It is important to not only recognize the importance of mentorship in surgical training, but it is also imperative to recognize the work of pioneering surgeons who paved the way for modern refractive surgeons. From the ancient methods of using gemstones or water for magnification, to the invention of spectacles for presbyopia in the 13th century, to the modern pioneers of corneal and intraocular surgery, the evolution of refractive techniques has accelerated over the last quarter of the 20th century (Table 1-4). Familiarity with the development, including the potential complications and advantages, of each technique provides the depth of understanding that allows the combination of techniques in bioptics. Many authors have previously written about the history of refractive surgery, and these sources can serve as excellent references.[5,8-9]

TEXT OBJECTIVES

For the experienced and transitioning surgeon, fellow, or resident, and the comanaging ophthalmologist or optometrist, this text provides a framework upon which to understand the causes, management, and avoidance of intraoperative and postoperative complications of LASIK. Prevention includes the principles of patient selection and counseling that will be discussed in Chapter 2, as well as an understanding of laser and microkeratome technologies as outlined in Chapter 3. Combinations of techniques (in the context of specific cases in which mixed enhancements and retreatments were performed) are discussed in Chapter 8 and Section II: Patient Examples.

As in any field of study, a framework for the understanding of a complex body of knowledge is essential. Refractive surgery is rapidly evolving and there are numerous journal articles, texts, and courses available. This text is designed to compliment available sources of information about LASIK techniques, and the authors remain committed to the philosophy of surgeon mentoring and fellowship training as key elements in refractive surgery training. With a combined experience at our five centers across Canada of over 37,000 LASIK procedures, the authors hope to continue the tradition of sharing knowledge and experiences with colleagues with the shared goal of providing the highest level of service to LASIK patients.

REFERENCES

1. Gimbel HV, Anderson Penno EE. LASIK: The Calgary experience. *Operative Techniques in Cataract and Refractive Surgery.* Dec 1999;2(4):172-176.
2. Sun R, Gimbel HV, Anderson Penno EE. Intraocular lens power calculation after corneal refractive surgery remains challenging. *Ophthalmology.* 2000;107(2):226-228.
3. Gimbel HV, Sun R, Kaye GB. Refractive error in cataract surgery after previous refractive surgery. *J Cataract Refract Surg.* 2000;26:142-144.
4. Gimbel HV, Sun R, Furlong MT, et al. Accuracy and predictability of intraocular lens power calculation in postoperative PRK eyes. *J Cataract Refract Surg.* 2000;26(8).
5. Gimbel HV, Anderson Penno EE. *Refractive Surgery: A Manual of Principles and Practice.* Thorofare, NJ: SLACK Incorporated; 2000.
6. Zaldivar R, Davidorf JM, Oscherow S. The intraocular contact lens. In: Buratto L, Brint SF, eds. *LASIK: Principles and Techniques.* Thorofare, NJ: SLACK Incorporated; 1997:401-413.
7. Güell JL, Vazquez M, Gris O, et al. Combined surgery to correct high myopia: Iris claw phakic intraocular lens and laser in situ keratomileusis. *J Refract Surg.* 1999;15:529-537.
8. Schimmelpfennig BH, Waring III GO. Development of refractive keratotomy in the nineteenth century. In: Waring III, GO, ed. *Refractive Keratotomy for Myopia and Astigmatism.* St. Louis, Mo: Mosby-Year Book; 1992:171-257.
9. Pallikaris I. Development of LASIK. In: Machat JJ, ed. *Excimer Laser Refractive Surgery: Practice and Principles.* Thorofare, NJ: SLACK Incorporated; 1986:268-298.

2

Patient Selection and Preoperative Assessment

Careful patient selection and thorough preoperative counseling is essential to avoiding complications and optimizing patient satisfaction following LASIK. As with any surgical procedure, LASIK begins with a thorough preoperative exam. It is essential that patients understand potential risks and have appropriate expectations prior to undergoing LASIK. Each patient should undergo a formal orientation process before surgery.

At our center, LASIK is offered to patients who are at least 18 years old and have had stable refractions for 2 years. The refractive criteria for performing LASIK varies depending on patient preference as well as surgeon experience. In a full-service refractive surgery practice such as ours, each patient is offered the choice of modality or combinations of modalities that suit their individual refraction situation. Our guidelines are outlined in Table 2-1. Generally, LASIK is strongly recommended over PRK for more than 7.00 D myopia. LASIK is recommended for all degrees of primary hyperopia.

PREOPERATIVE ASSESSMENT

Patients wearing contacts are asked to leave soft contact lenses out for at least 48 hours and leave hard contact lenses, including rigid gas permeable lenses, out for 2

Table 2-1
Refractive Surgical Guidelines

LASIK	• +6.00 to -1.00 D to >-10.00 D (upper range is dependent on pachymetry)
PRK	• +1.00 to -6.00 D
ISCRS	• -1.00 to -4.00 D
Phakic IOL	• Age is <50 years without cataract
	• Moderate to high myopia if LASIK is contraindicated (thin corneas) with anterior chamber depth of >3.00 mm
	• High hyperopia if anterior chamber depth is >2.75 mm
Toric IOL	• Cases have <1.50 D of astigmatism
Lensectomy	• Any patient with >2+ nuclear sclerosis
	• Any posterior subcapsular cataract or cortical changes
	• Age is >50 years with high hyperopia
AK	• ~ >2.00 D of astigmatism with spherical equivalent of +0.50 to -0.50 D can be used as primary surgery if patient not a candidate for other modalities
	• May be used as an enhancement technique or in combination with lensectomy or phakic IOL

Note: Individual cases may differ from above.

weeks prior to the preoperative assessment. Patients may then resume contact lens wear, but are also counseled to remove contact lenses 12 to 24 hours prior to surgery.

A complete ocular and medical history is obtained from all patients (Figure 2-1). The ocular history should specifically include any previous refractive surgery, any other previous ocular surgery, ocular injuries, and retinal history. A thorough medical history should include specific questions about collagen vascular disease, diabetes, and hormonal changes (such as pregnancy). Medications, both topical and systemic, and allergies should also be noted.

PATIENT EDUCATION AND COUNSELING

Group seminars are often offered to facilitate communication of basic anatomic information and surgical options available for the correction of refractive errors. Most patients find this quite helpful in the early stages of the decision process. At many centers, the preliminary history and counseling are done by ancillary staff rather than the surgeon. However, if this is done, it is critical that the surgeon have explicit guidelines for the staff to follow for the history and counseling of refractive patients. The surgeon must also review and complete the history and counseling in person.

Every patient is asked why he or she is interested in refractive surgery to assess motivations and expectations. For example, some patients may not be aware that if both eyes are corrected for distance there may be a need for reading glasses, or "readers," as they age. Presbyopes with mild myopia (~2.00 D) should be

```
┌────────────────────────────────────────────────────────────────────────────┐
│                                                                            │
│          GIMBEL EYE CENTRE - PATIENT HISTORY                               │
│                                                                            │
│                                Patient ID:                                 │
│                                                                            │
│                                Date of Birth:   /  /                       │
│    Calgary, AB                 Age:                                        │
│                                Health Care #:                              │
│                                                                            │
│    Phone #: (H) (   )   -          Campaign: CALGARY GEC                    │
│             (W)                                                            │
│                                OD: _____             │
│    Contact: _____  OH: _____       │
│      Phone:                        GP:                                     │
│    _____                                            │
└────────────────────────────────────────────────────────────────────────────┘
```

FAMILY HISTORY

	Yes	No		Yes	No
Glaucoma			Diabetes		
Cataracts			High Blood Pressure		
Lazy Eye			Heart Problems		
Retina Problems			Other:		
Blindness					

PATIENT HISTORY

	OD OS				
Glaucoma	[ ] [ ]	_____	Diabetes	_____	
Cataracts	[ ] [ ]	_____	High Blood Pressure	_____	
Lazy Eye	[ ] [ ]	_____	Heart Problems	_____	
Retina Problems	[ ] [ ]	_____	Asthma/Bronchitis	_____	
Dry Eye	[ ] [ ]	_____	Arthritis	_____	
Eye Infection	[ ] [ ]	_____	Keloid Scarring	_____	
Eye Injury	[ ] [ ]	_____	Pregnant/Lactating	_____	
Contact Lenses	[ ] [ ]	_____	Other:		
Cataract Sx	[ ] [ ]	_____			
EOM Surgery	[ ] [ ]	_____			

MEDICATIONS/ALLERGIES

Eye Medications being used: General Medications being used:

Allergies to Eye Medications: Other Allergies:

Occupation: _____   Dominant Eye: OD___ OS___ Alt___
Hobbies: _____   Age 1st Rx glasses prescribed ____
Decreased vision affects: Vision good & equal until age ____
        Work / Driving / Reading

/mjm/pathist.frm

Figure 2-1. Sample patient history form.

approached with care, because correction of both eyes for distance may lead to the immediate need for reading glasses postoperatively. These patients are generally used to seeing well at near without correction and may not realize that by having refractive surgery, they will be exchanging distance glasses for readers. This is particularly disturbing to patients who read for extended periods of time without glasses and women who discover they can no longer apply makeup without readers. It may be helpful to demonstrate this by having them read or look in the mirror through their current glasses or a trial frame.

Patients nearing presbyopic age and not yet wearing bifocals (in their late 30s and early 40s) should be forewarned that if both eyes are corrected for distance, then readers will likely be necessary by early to mid-40s—but may be needed sooner. Occasionally, a patient such as this will find that even though he or she was able to read through spectacles preoperatively, he or she requires reading glasses immediately postoperatively. This is due to the higher accommodative demand that results from a corneal plane correction.

Patients with amblyopia occasionally think that refractive surgery will improve the best corrected visual acuity (BCVA). A detailed discussion of the LASIK procedure including risks, benefits, and expectations should be undertaken with each patient prior to scheduling surgery, and special care should be taken when counseling presbyopes and near presbyopes.

Patients with inappropriate expectations should be identified preoperatively to avoid dissatisfaction after LASIK surgery is performed. A specific mention should be made regarding the possibility of glare, halos, and night vision difficulties; this is of particular importance in high corrections and in patients with large pupils (see Section 2, Patient Examples 24 and 25). One should also include the mention of retreatments, especially in cases where there may be a greater possibility that additional surgery will be necessary (eg, for patients with high astigmatism). This detailed discussion must include a comparison of the risks and benefits of PRK versus LASIK, as well as lensectomy with an IOL implant or phakic IOLs if those are appropriate options. Occasionally, patients may elect to cancel surgery after learning more about possible side effects of surgery (Figure 2-2). Finally, the surgeon should specifically ask if there are any additional questions that the patient may wish to have answered prior to surgery, and if he or she needs any explanation or has any questions regarding the informed consent they will be signing. Patients who are well informed and have appropriate expectations will be more satisfied with their refractive surgery experience overall.

All patients receive lensometry, auto refractometry, auto keratometry, manual keratometry, corneal topography (preferably elevation as well as Placedo disc technology), determination of eye dominance, visual acuity (VA) with and without correction, manifest and cycloplegic refraction with vertex measurements, pupil assessment in dim and bright light, stereopsis, intraocular pressure (IOP) measurements, pachymetry, notation of palpebral fissure measurements if narrow, horizontal white-to-white corneal diameter measurements, slit lamp exam, and dilated fundus exam. Lid abnormalities, such as ptosis, lid retraction, or lagophthalmos should be noted, as there may be a risk for postoperative flap dislocation or significant dry eye. Dry eye with SPK on an exam or a history of contact lens intolerance due to dry eye may indicate a high risk for significant dry eye postoperatively (see Patient Example 23). Dry eye is one of the most common causes of unhappiness, discomfort, and blurred vision postoperatively. Patients with these preoperative findings should be counseled that they are at high risk for this postoperative complication, and dryness may take up to 12 months to resolve.

A 36-year-old man in good health with a history of soft contact lens wear for 8 years presented for refractive surgery assessment.

Cycloplegic refraction was -7.25 -0.75 x 95, best corrected to 20/15-2 OD, and -7.50 -0.50 x 60 corrected 20 20/20-1 OS. The slit lamp and fundus exams were negative. The patient was noted to have pupils of 4 mm in normal light and 8 mm in dim light.

Just prior to surgery he was counseled that considering his large pupils in dim light, he would be more likely to experience night vision difficulty and may find this disabling. After this discussion, he elected to cancel LASIK surgery.

This example illustrates how the preoperative counseling should be tailored to the individual patient. In some cases such as this, the surgeon and patient may elect not to proceed with surgery. Forewarning of the increased risk may avoid patient dissatisfaction should a complication occur.

Figure 2-2. Large pupil, LASIK surgery canceled by patient.

Placement of punctal plugs preoperatively should be considered in these patients. If indicated, retinal drawings, specular microscopy, and A-scan are obtained. Computer-assisted medical records aid in quick access to information and allow records to be accessed for ongoing outcomes review (Figure 2-3).

As with all of the findings on the preoperative workup, any abnormalities on slit lamp or dilated funduscopic exam should be considered carefully. A common finding among refractive patients is a limbal vascular pannus due to long-standing contact lens use. While this is not a true complication of LASIK surgery, it may result in bleeding that can be a nuisance intraoperatively. Older patients with 20/25 or even 20/20 Snellen acuity who have early nuclear sclerosis should be made aware that refractive lensectomy with IOL implantation is another option for the correction of refractive errors. Patients with high myopia or evidence of any retinal pathology should have retinal drawings, and any findings on funduscopic exam should be discussed and referred for possible treatment.

Examples of important preoperative findings are outlined in Table 2-2. Often, careful attention to details of the preoperative history and workup will allow the surgeon to warn the patient that he or she is at a higher risk for a particular complication, to take special care during a particular point in the surgery to avoid complications, to suggest an alternative to LASIK (such as PRK, refractive lensectomy, or phakic IOL) or to recommend the patient not undergo refractive surgery.

DOCUMENTATION

Complete records are important for optimizing patient care, medicolegal reasons, and for outcomes analysis.

INFORMED CONSENT

To obtain informed consent, sufficient information must be given to the patient with regard to the nature and purpose of the proposed procedure or treatment, the expected outcome, the likelihood of success, the risk, the alternatives

```
REFRACTIVE CLINIC                                                    Page:  1
Print By: SP                    GECCGY Refractive Clinic
                                Refractive Assessment Only
ID:
Name:                                    Age:  46              Visit Date:
─────────────────────────────────────────────────────────────────────────────
                              TECHNICIAN:
─────────────────────────────────────────────────────────────────────────────
HISTORY: Interested in refractive sx.  Has attended seminar.  Pt not referred.
         Has worn soft c/l's x 18 yrs.  Only wears c/l's occasionally now due to
         extensive computer use.
         c/o problems with dryness with c/l's.  States she gets occasional eye
         infections from eye make-up.
         No other c/o.
O-MED ALLERGIES:
MOTIVATION FOR SX: 0
                   Want to be Free from Corrective Lens
Dominant Eye: Left eye
```

	RIGHT EYE	LEFT EYE
Ocular Medications:	No medications	No medications

```
Medications: None
MEDICATION ALLERGIES: NKA  (PEN. OK)
─────────────────────────────────────────────────────────────────────────────
Stereo: 40 seconds of arc              NPC: Good
Near Cover Test: Esophoria             Dist Cover Test: Appears Straight
Eye Color: Brown                       Ocular Motility: Within normal limits
─────────────────────────────────────────────────────────────────────────────
                 VASC: Count fingers at 3 meters    Count fingers at 3 meters
Distance Glasses Rx: -3.50 -1.00 x 13 ADD: 0.75     -3.75 -0.75 x 7 ADD: 0.75
                     Progressive addition lens      Progressive addition lens
                     Dec '97  cp                     Dec '97  cp
 Vision with Glasses: 20/20         6/ 6            20/20         6/ 6
                      +2                             +2
   Auto Refractometry: -3.50 -1.25 x 6              -3.75 -0.50 x 2
Manifest Refractomet: -3.25 -1.00 x 15              -3.75 -0.75 x 15
     Manifest VACC: 20/20           6/ 6            20/20         6/ 6
                    +2                               +2
Cycloplegic Refracto: -3.25 -1.00 x 13              -3.75 -0.75 x 10
   Cycloplegic VACC: 20/20          6/ 6            20/20         6/ 6
                     +3
─────────────────────────────────────────────────────────────────────────────
          Pachometry: 0.560mm                       0.565mm
                      Pach-Pen                       Pach-Pen
─────────────────────────────────────────────────────────────────────────────
 Manual Keratometry: 44.25 2 x 45.12 92             44.25 8 x 45.00 98
Auto Keratometry-Cen: 44.25 @ 179 45.00 @ 89        44.00 @ 4 45.25 @ 94
   Corneal Mapping: Technomed                       Technomed
─────────────────────────────────────────────────────────────────────────────
  Cornea Diameter: 12.00 mm                         12.00 mm
                   Using ARK                         Using ARK
                   cp                                cp
               AT: 14 @ 1549                         14 @ 1549
         AC Depth: Deep                              Deep
           Pupils: Light: 4.50 mm   Dim: 6.00 mm    Light: 4.50 mm   Dim: 6.00 mm
                   PERRL, No RAPD                    PERRL, No RAPD
  Drops instilled: Time: 1542                        Time: 1542
                   Mydriacyl 1.0% X 2                Mydriacyl 1.0% X 2
                   Time: 1547                        Time: 1547
                   Alcaine 0.5% drop and             Alcaine 0.5% drop and
                   Fluorescein dye                   Fluorescein dye
─────────────────────────────────────────────────────────────────────────────
Tech Comments: Discussed: pt's correction, PRK vs LASIK, risks and side effects,
               presbyopia, mono-vision.  Showed pt what mono-vision would be like
               through phoropter.  Encouraged pt to simulate mono-vision with c/l's.
─────────────────────────────────────────────────────────────────────────────
Examined by:          MD              Clinical Assistant:            COT
─────────────────────────────────────────────────────────────────────────────
      Conjunctiva: Quiet                            Quiet
          Cornea: Trace neovascularization          Trace neovascularization
            Lids: Lids & lashes clean               Lids & lashes clean
Anterior Chamber: Deep and quiet                    Deep and quiet
            Iris: Normal                            Normal
            Lens: Trace nuclear sclerosis           Trace nuclear sclerosis
                  through dilated                   through dilated pupil
                              — More —
```

Figure 2-3. Sample computer-assisted medical records.

Table 2-2
Preoperative Factors*

Motivations	• Verify appropriate motivations and expectations
Past eye history	• History of contact lens use (verify when last used) • History of dry eye • Previous ocular surgery (scleral buckle) or corneal injuries may predispose to poor exposure or suction failures • Prior history of steroid-induced ocular hypertension or medication allergies
Past medical history	• Collagen vascular diseases may pose a risk for melts • Hormonal status (pregnancy, breast-feeding) or diabetes may cause refractive instability
Medications	• Hormonal status, diabetes, or exogenous steroids may alter refraction • Systemic medications may induce mydriasis
Eye dominance	• If considering monovision, the dominant eye is generally corrected for distance
Age	• Care should be taken when counseling presbyopes or near presbyopes • Patients should be at least 18 years of age and caution should be taken in younger patients (early 20s) to verify a stable refraction
Refraction	• Cycloplegic refraction may reveal more hyperopia or less myopia, especially in younger patients • Discrepancy between Ks and refraction may indicate higher risk for undercorrection or overcorrection of astigmatism • Refraction should have been stable for 1 year prior to surgery
Pachymetry	• Must be adequate, especially important in high corrections
Manual keratometry	• Note overly steep or flat corneas, they may be prone to flap complications • Excessive flattening or steepening may produce poor quality of vision
IOP	• Ocular hypertension or glaucoma may be seen on refractive assessment. Patients should be counseled that corneal refractive surgery may alter IOP readings postoperatively
Pupil size	• Patients with large pupils (>6.5 mm in bright light, >7 mm in dim light) need to be forewarned of the possibility of night vision difficulties. Especially important in high corrections • Corneal surgery may not be advisable
Slit lamp exam	• *Lid abnormalities*—May predispose to poor exposure, which may be a risk for flap dislocation. Note early cataracts in presbyopes, lensectomy with IOL implant may be a better option • *Superficial punctate keratopathy*—These eyes are at risk for significant symptomatic dry eye for up to 1 year postoperatively

	Table 2-2 continued
	Preoperative Factors*
	• *Blepharitis*—These eyes may be at increased risk for infections or infiltrates
	• *Corneal dystrophies*—Patients may be predisposed to epithelial problems, may need phototherapeutic keratectomy (PTK)
Fundus	• All patients should have dilated exam, higher myopes and patients with prior history of retinal problems should have retinal drawings
	• Any pathology should be noted and referred for treatment if needed

*Note: The above are examples (not an exhaustive list) of factors that can be noted preoperatively and may allow the surgeon to either alter the LASIK technique slightly (eg, use a deeper cut), counsel the patient that they may be at increased risk for a complication, and/or cancel the surgery or suggest an alternative. *The surgeon must be vigilant when reviewing preoperative information and carefully consider all factors that may impact surgical outcome.*

to the procedure, the supporting information regarding those alternatives, and the effect of no treatment. While various tools for patient education and counseling can be used, including video or CD-ROM presentations, the surgeon must meet with the patient preoperatively to ensure there are no additional patient concerns or questions.

CONCLUSION

The surgeon must make a practice of carefully reviewing the results of the preoperative assessment with the goal of anticipating potential problems and avoiding complications. A more indepth discussion of factors predisposing to particular complications will be presented in the chapters to follow and in the Patient Examples in Section II.

COMANAGEMENT ISSUES FOR THE PRIMARY EYE CARE PROVIDER

Dennis A. Braun, OD

Optimizing the Comanaging Relationship

Ensuring continuity of care from the preoperative assessment through surgery and postoperative care requires effort on the part of both the surgery center and the referring practitioner. There are several strategies to optimize your relationship with your referral center. These and other issues in comanagement are covered in Chapter 6 of *Refractive Surgery: A Manual of Principles and Practice,* by H. Gimbel and E. Anderson Penno. Practices referring higher volumes of refractive surgery patients may want to invest in specialized equipment such as corneal topography or even pachymetry. At our center, a minimum of three postoperative visits are required after LASIK surgery. More visits may be required in the event of enhancement surgery.

Preoperative Assessment and Referrals

Patient selection and workup are covered in this chapter. A few topics require special emphasis to ensure the patient has a satisfactory outcome.

Careful attention should be paid to the measurement of pupil size in low light. This can be a difficult measurement in terms of accuracy and reliability, particularly if a simple pupil gauge is used for this purpose. Newer autorefractors have built-in pupil measurement options that work well if the autorefractor is situated in a setting where all the ambient illumination can be turned off. Another alternative is to use the telescopic alignment device on the visual field analyzer with the minimum illumination necessary to get a reading. The slit lamp can also be used for this purpose by quickly matching the dilated pupil size to the length of the slit as the slit is moved from shut to open.

In our experience, LASIK is most often canceled due to low pachymetry readings. There must be sufficient corneal thickness to allow for ablation zone diameters that will encompass the dilated pupil. If the patient presents with 7.0 mm pupils in dim light and a refraction >-8.00 D, you may want to caution the patient that scheduling surgery would be tentative pending adequate corneal thickness readings.

For presbyopic patients, a complete discussion of the impact of surgery on near vision should be undertaken. The option of monovision should be discussed for those patients who would wish to be as free from correction as possible. At our center, we prefer that a trial of monovision with contact lenses be undertaken preoperatively before considering this as a target correction. We rarely undercorrect by more than -1.25 D unless the patient has demonstrated an ability to tolerate a greater anisometropia in advance with contact lenses. For patients in their 50s, this degree of monovision may not be sufficient to allow them to read finer print, but they should be able to avoid needing a multifocal for intermediate vision by selecting monovision.

Referring practitioners would want to be vigilant for symptoms and signs of dry eyes in the preoperative assessment. If the patient is symptomatic, he or she should be alerted that proceeding with refractive surgery may make the symptoms worse. In contrast, patients experiencing dryness problems related to contact lens wear generally do better after refractive surgery. If blepharitis or meibomian dysfunction is a factor contributing to symptoms of dryness, this issue should be treated preoperatively with appropriate lid hygiene and antibiotic therapy.

Postoperative Comanagement of LASIK

Expected Clinical Findings

One day postoperative visit: Principle concerns for this visit include: confirming correct flap position, no interface inflammation, no macrowrinkles that require repositioning, and no infection. Normal findings include minor amounts of interface debris (usually consisting largely of metallic debris from the "wake" of the blade and fibers from sponges). Small microstriae may be evident on slit lamp retroillumination. Usually these do not impact on BCVA. If these striae are readily visible with retinoscopy, then consultation with the surgeon may be indicated. Retinoscopy is also useful in assessing the uniformity of the ablation pattern. A spot in the ablation pattern from a water spot on a mirror will be readily visible on retinoscopy as a dark opacity with surrounding distortion. Various degrees of surface superficial punctate keratitis (SPK) may be noted on this visit. Increased lubrication with Celluvisc (Allergan Inc, Markham, ON) or similar viscous lubricating agents is recommended. We do not routinely refract patients at 1 day postoperative. Autorefraction is usually sufficient at this point and a pinhole acuity may be taken if the uncorrected acuity is less than 20/40. Diffuse lamellar keratitis (DLK) should be referred back to the refractive surgery center on an urgent basis. In the event of a delay in this process the patient can be started on intensive topical steroid therapy every 1 to 2 hours and continue antibiotic cover.

One week postoperative visit: The cornea should be relatively clear and quiet at this point. The emphasis shifts toward the refractive outcome at this visit. Manifest refraction and keratometry (and corneal topography if available) are performed. Symptoms of dryness may be prominent, and glare and halos around lights will be maximal at this phase of recovery. Slit lamp findings may include mild SPK or be unremarkable with the flap in good position and interface debris remaining unchanged. Patients may notice a subconjunctival hemorrhage from the suction ring and need to be reassured that this will clear up shortly. Frequently, patients will exhibit an over-response at this visit with the anticipation of future regression toward the target refraction. Temporary reading glasses may be required for older myopes exhibiting an early postoperative hyperopic refraction. Any prescription eyewear should be delayed until refractive stability is achieved in 6 to 8 weeks.

One month postoperative visit: Regression of refraction should be evident now with the patient approximating the target refraction. If uncorrected acuity is reduced as a result of regression the patient may be disappointed, having experienced good vision in the early postoperative period. If vision is compromised sufficiently to disqualify the patient from driving, temporary correction may be required (usually disposable contact lenses or inexpensive single vision spectacle lenses) until the refraction stabilizes sufficiently to allow for retreatment surgery.

In a small minority of patients, epithelial ingrowth may be evident at this visit. (see Table 7-1). Minor amounts of ingrowth (<1.0 mm) can be monitored without treatment. If there is evidence of progression at the next postoperative visit the patient should be referred back to the attending surgeon.

Three month postoperative visit: Refraction is usually stable in the majority of cases at this visit. Exceptions include high myopes (>-8.00 D) and moderate hyperopes who may not be stable until 6 months postoperatively. Halos and glare at night will have diminished in most patients, possibly due to corneal remodeling, or more likely due to neural integration and adaptation. In a minority of patients, disabling glare and halos may persist. These patients can be advised that improvement of night vision can be see in some cases up to 12 months. Options for amelioration of this problem include: night-driving spectacles with a small degree of myopic correction (to stimulate accommodative miosis) with an anti-glare coating; parasympathomimetic drops (pilocarpine 0.5% gtts diluted in artificial tears to 0.25% or less) or sympatholytic drops such as RevEyes (Bausch & Lomb Surgical, Rochester, NY—not available in Canada) to produce a small amount of pupillary constriction; and zone enlargement surgery using a combination of hyperopic ablation with offsetting myopic ablation to expand the optical zone (this option would be restricted by the amount of stromal bed thickness remaining and risks jeopardizing what may be a good initial refractive outcome necessitating a third ablation).

Dryness issues should be either resolved or relatively minor at this point. However, some patients will have marked instability of their tear film, often accompanied by superficial punctate keratitis inferiorly or as an intrapalpebral band across the central cornea. The issue of nocturnal lagophthalmos should be addressed as a first step with nighttime occlusion (with tape or moisture chamber bubbles) as a diagnostic test and, if confirmed, bedtime application of bland ointment or other viscous lubricants. If dryness problems persist during the day even with the use of artificial tears and/or gels, then occlusion of the lower lacrimal puncta with silicone plugs would be indicated. Other measures to control this problem include sunglasses with side-shields to reduce the influence of wind-induced evaporation; Lacrisert (Merck Frosst, Kirkland, Quebec, Canada) ophthalmic inserts; increased ambient humidity in the home; or a course of tetracycline if there is meibomian dysfunction contributing to a poor tear film. Dryness may also continue to improve for up to 12 months postoperatively.

Long-Term After Care

Patients need to be made aware that regular eye examinations are necessary to ensure optimum ocular health after successful refractive surgery. Recommended annual or biennial examinations should be continued irrespective of the need for refractive correction.

3

Microkeratomes and Laser Systems

MICROKERATOME SYSTEMS

There are many different microkeratome systems available to today's refractive surgeon. Each has unique advantages, disadvantages, and learning curves. Regardless of the microkeratome used, the surgeon must have a complete understanding of its assembly and use. Practice handling the microkeratome in the wet lab prior to performing LASIK on patients is imperative. In addition, a thorough check should be made of the assembled microkeratome prior to each use. Examples of inspection points for the Automated Corneal Shaper (ACS) and Hansatome are outlined in Table 3-1. This should be done by the scrub nurse and/or the surgeon. Some surgeons have made the analogy to a pilot's pre-flight check list done prior to each flight. This minimizes the risk of mechanical failure due to things, such as debris on the tracks or an improperly seated blade. The following is an overview of the most commonly used microkeratome systems presented by surgeons with significant experience with their respective microkeratome.

Table 3-1
Inspection Points

ACS	• Confirm depth plate (eg, 160 or 180 µ) • Check for proper insertion of depth plate. Check that it is present and fully inserted • Check for advancement of stopper • Check that all parts are snug: cuff, motor head, depth plate, power cords, suction tubing, suction handle • Check blade under a microscope • Visually inspect gears and manually check for freedom of movement • Visually confirm blade movement • Inspect suction ring, clear any debris or BSS crystals • Visually verify suction port is open • Seat microkeratome on suction ring and verify full microkeratome pass (forward and reverse) prior to placing on the eye • Confirm depth of head (eg, 160 or 180 µ) • Confirm right or left eye assembly
Hansatome	• Inspect blade under microscope • Visually inspect keratome head, check gears for debris • Manually confirm gears move freely • Check that the motor head is snugly seated • Visually confirm blade movement • Visually inspect suction ring, clear any debris or BSS crystals from tracks • Visually verify suction port is open • Seat microkeratome on suction ring and verify full microkeratome pass (forward and reverse) prior to placing on the eye

THE CHIRON HANSATOME ACS AND CHIRON ACS (BAUSCH & LOMB, ROCHESTER, NY)

Nader G. Iskander, MD, Diplomate ABO, and N. Timothy Peters, MD

The Chiron Hansatome

The majority of LASIK cases at our center have been done with the Chiron Hansatome (Figure 3-1). The Hansatome has the advantage of creating a superior hinge (Figure 3-2). This superior location means that the natural action of the upper lid does not pose a risk for dislocating the flap. The flap created by the Hansatome is also somewhat larger, and therefore advantageous for the expanded zones used in hyperopic corrections and in low myopes with large pupils. In addition, this microkeratome system is less prone to interference of the lid or drapes as compared to the ACS during the microkeratome pass due to the elevation and location of the track (Figure 3-3). If there is an obstruction from the speculum or eyelid, the motor has more torque to overcome this resistance. Some surgeons may find that it is easier to seat the Hansatome microkeratome head onto the suction ring due to the presence of a peg on one side and a single track on the other (Figures 3-3 and 3-4). The creation of a larger flap may have the

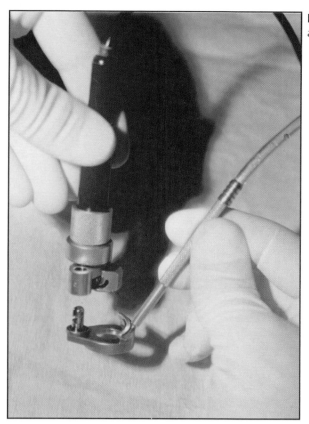

Figure 3-1. Chiron Hansatome and its suction ring.

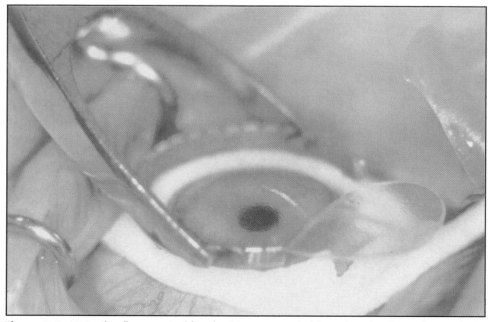

Figure 3-2. Note the flap created by the Hansatome is hinged and reflected superiorly.

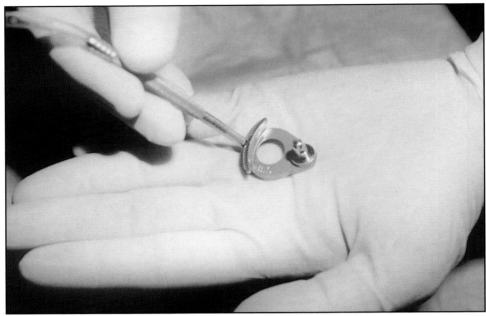

Figure 3-3. Note the Hansatome track is elevated, which keeps it out of the way of drapes and lid speculum.

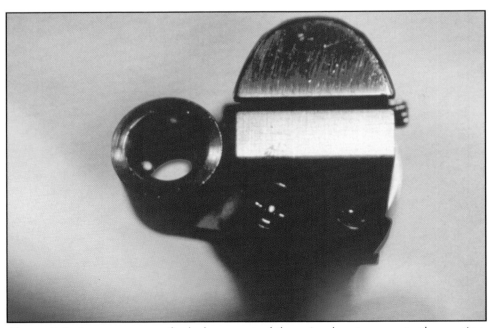

Figure 3-4. Some surgeons find placement of the microkeratome onto the suction ring easier with the Hansatome. The single hole on the microkeratome head fits onto the single peg on the suction ring (see Figure 3-3).

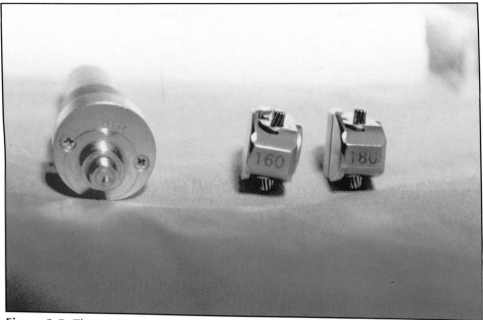

Figure 3-5. The 160-µ and 180-µ heads of the Hansatome.

disadvantage of being more prone to bleeding if there is a superficial corneal pannus or in eyes with small corneas. However, the Hansatome allows the creation of either an 8.5 mm or 9.5 mm flap by the use of different size suction rings. Another advantage to the Hansatome is the absence of removable depth plates. The Hansatome has separate microkeratome heads for the 160 µ and 180 µ depth (Figure 3-5). This eliminates the risk of improper placement or failure to place the depth plate, which would lead to corneal perforation

The Chiron ACS

The Chiron ACS was originally developed for use in ALK (Figures 3-6a and b). With this microkeratome, care should be taken to ensure that the stopper on the sleeve is properly advanced to avoid the creation of free caps. One of the difficulties novice surgeons face with this microkeratome is properly seating the microkeratome head onto the tracks of the suction ring. Some surgeons may find that practicing this with their eyes closed is helpful in learning tactile clues to augment visual clues.

Another feature of the ACS is the interchangeable spacer (a 160 µ or 180 µ spacer is generally used for creating the flap during the LASIK procedure, see Figure 3-7). If this spacer is not placed or is incompletely inserted prior to use, the cut will perforate the cornea and enter the anterior chamber. Therefore, care must be taken to check the position of the spacer since it is possible to operate the microkeratome even if the spacer is not completely seated. This will result in a deeper cut then is indicated on the spacer (Figure 3-8). A more common problem

Figure 3-6a. Fully assembled ACS. (Reprinted with permission from Gimbel HV, Anderson Penno EE. *LASIK Complications: Prevention and Management.* Thorofare, NJ: SLACK Incorporated, 1999.)

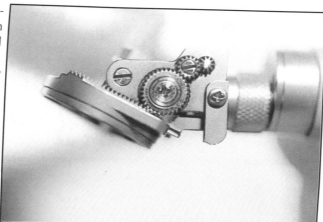

Figure 3-6b. ACS (shown at a different angle) illustrating the fully assembled microkeratome with the adjustable stopper located superiorly for the right eye. (Reprinted with permission from Gimbel HV, Anderson Penno EE. *LASIK Complications: Prevention and Management.* Thorofare, NJ: SLACK Incorporated, 1999.)

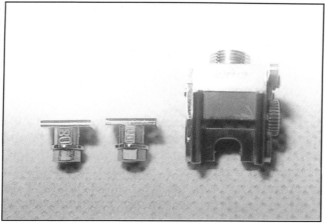

Figure 3-7. 160-µ and 180-µ spacers of the ACS. These are two of the available depth plates that must be inserted fully into the microkeratome head prior to use. (Reprinted with permission from Gimbel HV, Anderson Penno EE. *LASIK Complications: Prevention and Management.* Thorofare, NJ: SLACK Incorporated, 1999.)

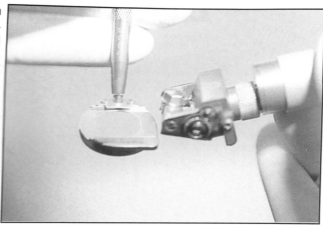

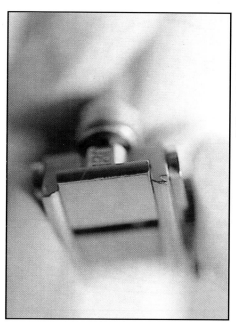

Figure 3-8. This photo illustrates partial insertion of the 180-μ depth plate into the ACS microkeratome head. This plate must be fully advanced to avoid corneal perforation. (Reprinted with permission from Gimbel HV, Anderson Penno EE. *LASIK Complications: Prevention and Management.* Thorofare, NJ: SLACK Incorporated, 1999.)

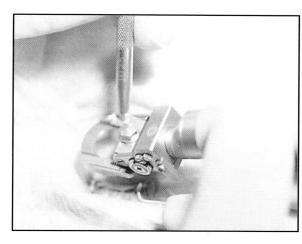

Figure 3-9. Microkeratome pass on the right eye. This figure illustrates the need for special attention with regard to interference of the microkeratome from the upper lid and drapes when using the ACS on the right eye. In this situation, the adjustable stopper is located superiorly; whereas, when performing the microkeratome pass on the left eye, the stopper is located inferiorly (where there is less likely to be interference from the lid or drapes). (Reprinted with permission from Gimbel HV, Anderson Penno EE. *LASIK Complications: Prevention and Management.* Thorofare, NJ: SLACK Incorporated, 1999.)

encountered is that of inadequate exposure, with the drapes or lid interfering with the microkeratome pass, resulting in an incomplete pass. Incomplete passes with the Chiron ACS may be more likely when performing LASIK on the right eye, due to the location of the stopper. When used on the right eye, the stopper is located superiorly and is more likely to catch on the upper lid, speculum, or drape (Figure 3-9).

Analysis of the first 1000 LASIK cases of one surgeon indicate that when using the ACS, very steep corneas should probably be cut deeper than 160 μ and very flat corneas should have the stopper set for a shorter pass or larger hinge.

Alternatively, the flap could be cut with the Chiron Hansatome or with a micro-keratome that has different suction rings for different eye shapes. Another alternative for flat corneas is to visually control the stop of the cut; however, this takes practice and even experienced surgeons can create a free cap using this method.

MORIA/MICROTECH MICROKERATOMES (DOYLESTOWN, PA)

Ashley Behrens, MD, Lee H. Novick, MD, Lawrence Chao, MD, and Roy S. Chuck, MD, PhD

Three microkeratome models especially designed for LASIK surgery are currently available from Moria/Microtech: LSK One, One disposable, and Carriazo-Barraquer.

Common Features

These systems have many common features. The three systems utilize the latest control unit model, "Evolution II." The former control unit models only work with the LSK One-One disposable system.

Five different sizes of suction rings are available (H, -1, 0, +1, +2), to obtain approximate flap sizes according to keratometry reading nomograms. These numbers reveal the thickness of the suction ring plate, which is related to the amount of exposed cornea desired. The thinnest (H, "Hyperopic") ring exposes the highest amount of cornea to the microkeratome; and therefore, flaps are the largest possible. The thickest ring (+2) exposes the least amount of cornea; and therefore, flaps are the smallest possible.

These microkeratomes utilize the oscillating blade principle. Blades are oriented at 25 degrees to the cut plane. Single-use stainless steel blades are not interchangeable. LSK One blades will not fit in the Carriazo-Barraquer head, and vice versa. The One disposable heads have their own blade already installed.

Evolution II Control Unit

Provided with two pumps (second as reserve pump to maintain the suction in case of suction loss during the procedure), a nitrogen gas regulator, and a rechargeable battery to prevent electrical power-induced fluctuations on the suction. The console performs a self-test to detect malfunctioning. This test should be run before each case. A low-vacuum button allows the surgeon to maintain the suction ring as a fixation device after the keratectomy.

LSK One Microkeratome

This is the traditional microkeratome from Moria/Microtech. Based on the Barraquer-Krumeich-Swinger principle, it has a manually guided hand piece consisting of a turbine and a metal head. The hand piece is connected to the control unit through a gas hose.

Microkeratome Head

This was the first "single-piece" microkeratome head introduced to the market, with a predetermined thickness number identified on the metal head surface. The number is related to the distance between the cutting edge of the blade and the applanation plate of the head. It does not indicate the actual intended flap thickness. Three heads are available: 100 μ, 130 μ and 160 μ, to obtain approximately 130 μ, 160 μ and 180 μ thick flaps respectively. A new head to obtain 100 μ thick flaps will be available for high myopic ablations.

Dovetails are placed on both sides of the microkeratome head to match with the tracks at the suction ring. They should be clean at all times to guarantee a smooth translation of the head during the keratome pass. A stop ring with four different numbers is provided, to be coupled with the head before attachment to the turbine. It prevents the full pass of the microkeratome across the suction ring, allowing the creation of a hinged flap.

Blades should be inserted from one side in the orientation required at the receptacle. Any contact with the cutting edge should be avoided; the posterior zone of the blade should then be used as a point of contact when performing the procedure.

Heads should be cleaned with a nonabrasive liquid soap and a soft toothbrush after each use, then rinsed and carefully dried with air.

Turbine

A nitrogen gas driven turbine imparts an oscillation rate of 15,000 osc/min to the blade. The turbine surface may be wiped with alcohol after use for cleaning.

Advantages

- A single microkeratome head solves problems of using separate plates, saving assembly time and virtually avoiding the most feared complication of lamellar surgery: corneal perforation.
- Manual translation of the microkeratome allows more control of the translation speed.
- The flap is exposed and clearly observed during the keratectomy.
- Two-button foot pedal makes the procedure simpler.
- High oscillation blade rate tends to perform smoother cuts.
- One-step removal/insertion of the blade.

Disadvantages

- Translation of the microkeratome head across the suction requires some experience to get used to control the ideal plane correlation (vertical/horizontal) through the pass.
- Irregular speeds or inadvertent translation stops produce undesired surface ridges.
- Requires nitrogen gas to activate the turbine.

One Disposable Microkeratome

This microkeratome uses the same turbine and control unit as the LSK One. Basic differences lie in the materials of the head and suction ring, which are plastic instead of metal. The blades come already assembled in the transparent plastic head, and the suction ring has two different tubes on each side to apply the vacuum.

Advantages and disadvantages are similar to those already described with the LSK One. The difference in weight between both instruments and the properties of the plastic materials introduce some changes in the instrument handling. If the surgeon is familiar with the LSK One system, we believe that these differences in the disposable variant should be identified by the surgeon before using it on his or her first patient.

Carriazo-Barraquer Microkeratome

This is the most recent model in the market from Moria/Microtech, developed by Dr. César Carriazo and Dr. Jose Ignacio Barraquer. An interesting pivoting head change in the translation principle has been added to this system. The possibility of using two different turbines, an electric and a nitrogen gas driven, is also available.

Microkeratome Head

The metal heads in this unit are redesigned to receive the vertically oriented turbine. The insertion of the blades is similar to LSK One; it must match the orientation of the receptacle on one side. Similar care should be taken when inserting the blades to avoid touching the cutting edge with other surfaces. Three different heads are available: 100 μ, 130 μ, and 160 μ.

In order to pass the microkeratome over the corneal surface after placing the suction ring, the head should be attached to the turbine. A peripheral axle is present on one side of the suction ring, where the head is coupled. It is provided either with gears (in case an automated pass is desired) or a simple flat surface (when the manual translation is preferred). On the opposite side of this axle, circular shaped tracks to maintain the microkeratome dovetail in place are present. Another variant possible with this device is to position the flap hinge in the most convenient location. This can be oriented by a mark on one side of the suction ring. No stop rings are necessary, since it is included in the suction ring itself.

The same instructions used with the LSK One should be followed to clean the head.

Turbine

Two different types of turbine are offered with this instrument. A 12,000 osc/min electric motor driven turbine with capabilities of both manual and automated pass of the head across the suction ring, and a 15,000 osc/min nitrogen gas driven turbine with only manual pass capabilities. Alcohol may be used to wipe the electric turbine, and the nitrogen turbine should be cleaned following the same parameters mentioned in the LSK One section.

Advantages

- Head translation is easier to perform using the manual version, especially for beginners.
- Variable hinge position, which may be helpful in astigmatic corrections, where a larger diameter for the astigmatic correction is necessary to avoid the hinge.
- One-step head installation; no need for stop rings.

Table 3-2
Excimer Laser Types

Broadbeam	*Scanning Slit*	*Flying Spot*
Summit: Excimed, Omni-med, Apex	**Aesculap-Meditec:** Meditec Mel 60	**Autonomous Technologies:** Tracker PRK
Excimer: SVS	**Apex Plus Nidek:** EC-5000	**LaserSight:** Compak-200 Mini
VISX: 20/20 B, Model B, 20/15 (Taunton), Star		**Chiron Technolas:** Keracor 117, Keracor 217
Chiron Technolas: Keracor 116		**Novatec:** Light blade (nonexcimer)
Coherent Schwind: Keratome I/II		**Kera Technology:** ISO beam

(Reprinted with permission from Gimbel HV, Anderson Penno EE. LASIK Complications: Prevention and Management. Thorofare, NJ: SLACK Incorporated, 1999.)

- Larger flaps possible (useful for hyperopic corrections).
- High oscillation rate with smoother cut surfaces.

Disadvantages

- Thicker flaps than expected (compared to LSK One using the same head numbers) have been reported.
- Flap hinge is usually smaller, which theoretically diminishes flap stability.
- Visibility of the flap during keratectomy is hindered.
- Two button (for microkeratome translation), one button (for vacuum) foot pedals make procedure slightly more demanding compared to LSK One.

LASER TECHNOLOGY

Laser type and software characteristics also influence the complications that may be encountered. Currently, there are several manufacturers of excimer lasers worldwide; these fall into three types: broadbeam, scanning slit, and flying spot (Table 3-2). Each laser has particular characteristics with regard to beam shaping and homogeneity, beam size and energy, and optical zone size; each laser also varies with regard to astigmatic and hyperopic correction capabilities (Tables 3-3a and b). In general, laser hardware and software have undergone frequent modifications aimed at improving beam characteristics and ablation patterns. Just as a thorough understanding of the microkeratome is necessary, the surgeon should be familiar with the salient features of the laser system in use. In the United States (as of early 2000), the broadbeam systems by VISX and Summit Technology are currently approved by the Food and Drug Adminisatration (FDA) for treatment of myopia, astigmatism, and hyperopia. Other laser systems like Nidek, Technolas, Autonomous, and LaserSight are only approved for some degrees of myopia and astigmatism.

Since 1988, the authors have had experience with a variety of broadbeam and scanning lasers. Over the past several years we have used the Summit ExciMed

Table 3-3a

Excimer Laser System Features

Eyetracker	Fluence (mJ/cm2)	Maximum Pulse Frequency	Maximum Pulse Area
None: Summit, VISX, Aesculap-Meditec, LaserSight, Kera Technology	100 Novatec	6 VISX	Transition zone 2x 9.0 mm; Optical zone 7.5 mm (hyperopia optical zone $\leq$5.0 mm)
Active: Autonomous Technologies, Chiron Technolas, Novatec, Nidek (optional)	130 Chiron Technolas	10 Summit	1.5 x 10 mm Aesculap-Meditec
Passive: Coherent Schwind	150 Kera Technology	10 to 50 Chiron Technolas	<1 mm Autonomous Technologies, LaserSight, Novatec, Kera Technology
	160 VISX	13 Coherent Schwind	1 to 2 mm Chiron
	180 Autonomous Technologies, Summit, Nidek	20 Aesculap-Meditec	6.5 mm Summit
	250 Aesculap-Meditec	30 Nidek	7.0 mm Chiron
	Variable LaserSight (160 to 300), Coherent Schwind (<250)	100 LaserSight, Autonomous Technologies	8.0 mm VISX, Coherent Schwind
		>200	
		400 Kera Technology	

(Reprinted with permission from Gimbel HV, Anderson Penno EE. LASIK Complications: Prevention and Management. Thorofare, NJ: SLACK Incorporated, 1999.)

Table 3-3b

Excimer Laser Myopic/Hyperopic Patterns

Laser Type	Myopic	Hyperopic	Astigmatic
Summit	Iris diaphragm or erodible mask	Emphasis erodible mask	Erodible mask
VISX	Iris diaphragm	Rotating scanning slit	Rotatable slit, iris diaphragm
Chiron (broadbeam)	Iris diaphragm	Annular scanning spot	Linear scanning
Chiron (scanning beam)	Spiral random scanning spot, scanning spot using plano scan algorithms	Meridonal scanning, annular scanning spot	Meridonal scanning
Coherent Schwind	Enlarging circular apertures	Annular apertures	Enlarging oval apertures
Aesculap-Meditec	Rotating eye mask	Rotating inverse eye mask	Rotating eye mask
Nidek	Iris diaphragm scanning slit	Annular scanning slit beams rotating	Rotatable scanning slit
Autonomous Technologies	Spiral scanning	Annular scanning	Meridonal scanning
LaserSight	Rotating linear scanning spot	Annular scanning spot	Meridonal scanning
Novatec	Spiral scanning spot	Annular scanning spot	Annular and elliptical scanning spot
Kera Technology	Two fractal scanning spot	Two fractal scanning spot	Two fractal scanning spot

(Reprinted with permission from Gimbel HV, Anderson Penno EE. LASIK Complications: Prevention and Management. Thorofare, NJ: SLACK Incorporated, 1999.)

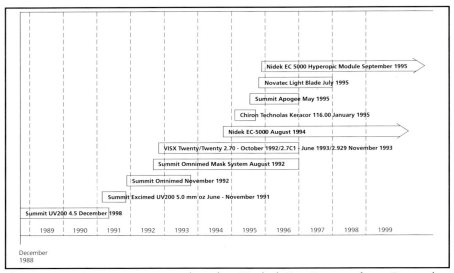

Figure 3-10. Laser systems used at the Gimbel Eye Centres from December 1988 to 1999. (Reprinted with permission from Gimbel HV, Anderson Penno EE. *Refractive Surgery: A Manual of Principles.* Thorofare, NJ: SLACK Incorporated, 2000.)

UV 200 4.5 mm, Summit ExciMed UV 200 6.0 mm (Summit Technology, Inc, Waltham, Mass), Summit OmniMed (APEX), Summit Apogee (APEX Plus), VISX Twenty/Twenty (software version 2.70, 2.7 Cl, and 2.92) (VISX, Inc., Santa Clara, Calif), Chiron Technolas Keracor 116, Novatec LightBlade (Novatec, Carlsbad, Calif), and Nidek EC-5000 (Nidek Co, Ltd, Gamagori, Japan) (Figure 3-10). Currently, virtually all LASIK and PRK at our centers are done with the Nidek EC-5000 scanning slit delivery system.

Our experience indicates that broadbeam delivery systems have a higher incidence of central islands and haze than occurs with the scanning slit system. In the past, central islands with the VISX 20/20 B and STAAR have been reported to be approximately 18%.[1] This has resulted in the development of anti-island software. With changes in delivery systems, techniques, and software, current estimates are that central islands occur in less than 4% of PRK cases.[2] According to Machat, central islands are the most common topographical abnormality encountered postoperatively in LASIK patients when a broadbeam laser system is used.[3] Factors other than laser type, such as slow re-epithelialization after PRK and the presence of fluid on the surface of the stromal bed, also may influence central island formation. Central island formation is extremely rare following treatment with scanning slit or flying spot systems.

Haze is uncommon following LASIK as compared to PRK, possibly due to the presence of an intact Bowman's membrane.[4] The formation of haze may be related to the quality of the surface created by the particular laser; the rougher surface created by the broadbeam iris diaphragm systems may lead to a higher incidence of haze.[5]

In addition to the characteristics of the particular laser system that affect the ablation, there are differences in ergonomics of the various laser systems. Fixation

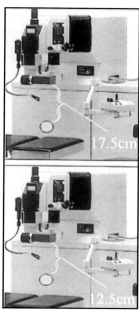

Figure 3-11. This figure illustrates the variety of working distances that may be obtained depending on the design of the laser. At our center, one laser has a working distance of 17.5 cm, and the other has a working distance of 12.5 cm. This distance is of concern in particular when using vertically oriented microkeratomes. (Reprinted with permission from Gimbel HV, Anderson Penno EE. *LASIK Complications: Prevention and Management.* Thorofare, NJ: SLACK Incorporated, 1999.)

patterns vary between laser systems and it is helpful for the surgeon to be familiar with the particular features so that detailed instructions can be given to the patient to enhance fixation. Some systems have a chair that locks into position and aids in patient positioning (of particular importance in astigmatic corrections). The way that patients can be positioned will also vary from system to system. Furthermore, working distances will be different depending on the viewing system in use (Figure 3-11). This becomes important in performing LASIK because of the need for suction ring and microkeratome placement.

The following is an overview of the most commonly used excimer laser systems presented by surgeons with significant experience with their respective lasers.

Nidek EC 5000
N. Timothy Peters, MD, and Nader G. Iskander, MD, Diplomate ABO

The Nidek EC 5000 is a scanning slit laser that operates by creating an excited dimmer of argon and fluorine gases. The pulse duration is 10 to 25 nanoseconds, and the repetition rate ranges from 5 to 50 Hz. There is also a long gas life—to a maximum of 80,000 shots within 8 hours after filling the laser. The aiming beam is a diode laser that projects a red target at a wavelength of 630 to 680 nm. There is a revolving turret magnification system ranging from 4x to 25x. This laser is widely in use throughout the world and has recently been approved for the treatment of mild and moderate myopia and astigmatism in the United States.

The Nidek has a control panel that the surgeon may operate with one hand (Figure 3-12). This panel can adjust the illumination, aiming, and focusing of the laser. These items can also be controlled with a foot pedal, which then frees both the surgeon's hands for use during the procedure (Figure 3-13).

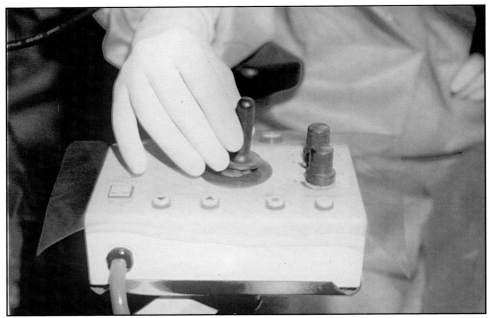

Figure 3-12. Nidek hand control panel for focusing in the x-y-z axis, aiming, and illumination control.

Figure 3-13. Nidek foot pedal for focusing and aiming.

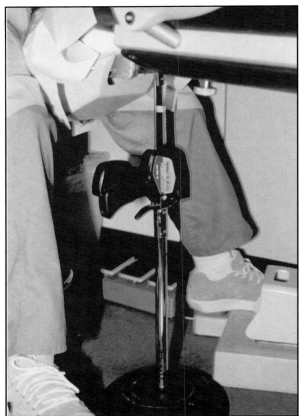

There are two slit beams inclined at 35 degrees projected onto the cornea. When these beams are superimposed, the laser is perfectly focused. These beams are also excellent for use at the conclusion of the case to inspect the interface under high magnification for interface debris and flap wrinkles.

The Nidek should be operated in a temperature range from 59° to 77°F, with a noncondensing humidity ranging from 0 to 70%.

The following are examples of nomograms (Note: nomograms need to be customized to surgical center and surgeon):

Myopia Nomogram

OZ	TZ	LASIK %	Cylinder Correction %
5.5	7.0	86 (84 if age > 45)	35
6.0	7.0	86 (82 if age > 45)	40
6.5	7.0	84 (80 if age > 45)	45
6.5	7.5	82 (78 if age > 45)	50

The cylinder correction has historically been subtracted from the sphere component prior to using the adjustment factor. In our newer algorithms, the cylinder correction is subtracted from the adjusted sphere; eg, a preoperative refraction of -5.00 -1.00 x 180° treated with a 6.5 mm OZ and a 7.0 mm TZ will be adjusted as follows:

$$-5.00 \times 84\% = \quad -4.20 \text{ D}$$
$$\underline{-1.00 \times 45\% = \quad 0.45 \text{ D}}$$
$$-3.75 \text{ D}$$

Therefore, you can program the laser for -3.75 -1.00 x 180°.

Hyperopia Nomogram

OZ	TZ	LASIK %	Cylinder Correction %
5.5	9.0	100	35

Phototherapeutic keratectomy (PTK) smoothing of 2 microns at 8.0 mm is performed with all hyperopic corrections—after the completion of the refractive laser treatments (see Chapter 9).

Ranges of Correction

Myopia	- 1.00 to -16.00
Hyperopia	+ 1.00 to + 7.00
Astigmatism	1.00 to 7.00

The following are our outcomes using the Nidek EC-5000 laser

1st Treatment			With Enhancement	
Amt. of correction	20/20 or Better	20/40 or Better	20/20 or Better	20/40 or Better
+4.01 to +7.00	68%	90%	80%	90%
+2.01 to +4.00	70%	95%	85%	95%
+0.50 to +2.00	80%	95%	90%	98%
0	-	-	-	-
-0.50 to -2.00	87%	96%	95%	98%
-2.01 to -4.00	83%	97%	92%	97%
-4.01 to -6.00	83%	95%	92%	97%
-6.01 to -8.00	77%	94%	90%	94%
-8.01 to -10.0	75%	94%	90%	94%
-10.01 to -12.0	75%	93%	90%	93%
-12.01 to -14.0	75%	91%	88%	93%
-14.01 to -16.0	75%	90%	83%	93%

Treatment Zones

The Nidek-EC 5000 offers a variety of optical zones and transitional zones. The optical zones are 5.5 mm for hyperopia and range between 5.5 and 6.5 mm for myopia. The transitional zones are 7.5 and 9.0 mm for hyperopia, and they range between 6.0 mm and 9.0 mm for myopia.

The Nidek is a very ergonomically friendly laser, and we have achieved excellent results with our current nomogram. We feel that with a minimal amount of practice, a surgeon can quickly become comfortable with the operating characteristics of the Nidek EC-5000.

Upcoming Modifications

Custom corneal ablation software is currently being launched by NIDEK. The first prototype will be tested in our center in the spring of 2000. It is expected that this will be an additional tool in treating decentration, and asymmetric or irregular astigmatism.

VISX STAAR S2 EXCIMER LASER (VISX, INC, SANTA CLARA, CALIF)

Lee H. Novick, MD, Ashley Behrens, MD, Lawrence Chao, MD, and Roy S. Chuck, MD, PhD

The VISX Staar S2 excimer laser system is a fourth generation 193 nm argon fluorine-based system widely used throughout the United States. Often considered to be a broadbeam laser, the Staar S2 institutes a sophisticated system to create a seven-beam scanning system. Use of this system requires user certification from VISX, as well as a vision card key system.

The laser beam delivery system consists of a beam rotator for temporal integration, a spatial integrator, and a beam shaping device that contains an iris diaphragm and rotating slit blades. This consists of 0.6 to 6.0 mm slit and a 2.0 to 6.5 mm circle. The modified broadbeam delivery system produces a combination of seven beams, which are delivered to the cornea in unison. This SmoothScan technology produces a highly regular ablation profile.

The laser has a simple and elegant design with basic controls. A single joystick is used for alignment, which moves the patient chair and not the laser. Control panel buttons are arranged in a mirror-like fashion on each side of the joystick. This allows the operator to adjust the ring and oblique illumination as well as a projected reticle (that can be removed for enhanced microscopy) for alignment. A bright red LED light is provided for patient fixation. A Leica MS microscope is a standard part of the laser, which allows for adjusting to three different magnification levels. A single aerosol aspirator can be swiveled into the in use and out of use positions to create extra space for lamellar sections underneath the laser using a microkeratome system of the surgeon's choice.

An IBM-compatible computer is utilized for the computer interface, and a write once read many (WORM) vision key card is provided to allow compilation and storage of patient data. The laser monitor allows a nicely organized windows-based screen of treatment options and data to be displayed and entered. The VISX S2 has numerous treatment and setting screens, which allows for adjustment of various parameters. A variable repetition rate is one of these options as well as an enhanced treatment zone up to 6.5 mm myopic and 9.5 mm hyperopic. System defaults are readily available, and warning screens are numerous for information omitted or out of treatment parameter zones. A printout of data entered and treatment parameters are readily available after treatment.

System calibration is important. Complete calibration is required at the start of each day when the laser is turned on, as well as a myopic -4.00 sphere calibration after three treatments. Laser operator confirmation is needed to verify a proprietary PMMA plastic card, which is cut and examined under a lensometer. Laser fluence is set prior to each treatment and if parameters are not met, automatic adjustments are made.

Treatment is initiated by a foot pedal, which controls the delivery of the ablation. The aspirating tube must be engaged in the down position and the patient chair locked for a blinking reticule to become solid. Ablation can be easily stopped by removal of the surgeon's foot from the pedal. An emergency stop button is also available.

There are few weak points of the VISX Staar S2. Illumination is good, but slit illumination for viewing the interface after the procedure is not available. The need for argon and fluorine gases is disadvantageous secondary to the toxic nature of fluorine, as well as the relatively high costs of these gases. High voltage is generated and flammable precautions must not be overlooked. There are recommended ranges of temperature and humidity for treatment, but no known adjustment is available for variables in these conditions. Currently, an eye tracking mode is not available. A well-placed gentian violet mark on the peripheral cornea is prudent prior to treatment to prevent intraoperative incyclotorsion or excyclotorsion.

At present, the largest myopic treatment zone is limited to 6.5 mm. Hyperopia with astigmatism cannot be treated simultaneously. Treatment nomograms are readily available.

FDA approval has been obtained at the time of this writing for myopia, hyperopia, and astigmatism. Astigmatism is treated via a slit/iris diaphragm with no disposable mask needed.

Specifications of the VISX Staar S2 Excimer Laser

Dimensions (WxDxH) Wt.	Wavelength Gas	Pulse Frequency	Fluence	Input Voltages
80x50x59 in 1600 lbs.	193 nm ArF	2 to 10 Hz	160mJ/cm²	Volts: 220 Amps: 30 Hz: 50 to 60

Cooling System	Pulse Area	Eye Tracker	FDA approval Treatment uses
Internal Water cooling	6.0 mm zone 6.5 mm zone	N/A	Low/Mod/High Myopia +6.00 D astigmatism Hyperopia -1.00-6.00 D Without astigmatism

THE SUMMIT APEX PLUS (SUMMIT TECHNOLOGY, INC, WALTHAM, MASS)

Daniel S. Durrie, MD, and Trent L. VandeGarde, MD

The Summit Apex Plus is a broadbeam laser that is capable of treating a wide range of refractive errors. It uses a combination of an expanding iris diaphragm and erodable discs. This laser has some particular advantages in the treatment of hyperopia. There have been significant improvements in this laser system with the addition of a recent upgrade package. Although the Summit Apex Plus is an easy laser to use, there are some key points to remember in order to avoid problems when treating patients.

The Summit Apex Plus has a fluence of 180 mJ/cm and a pulse frequency of 10 Hz. It has a maximum ablation diameter of 6.5 mm that extends to 9.5 mm when using the Axicon lens during hyperopic ablations. This laser does not have an eye tracker.

The Summit Apex Plus uses a combination of an expandable iris diaphragm and erodable polymethylmethacrylate (PMMA) discs to perform ablations. Myopic corrections can be performed with either the expanding iris diaphragm or an erodable disc. Hyperopia and astigmatism, however, must be performed using the discs. The ablations performed with the discs leave a very smooth stromal surface. The current approved myopia treatment range is from 0 to -14 D with astigmatism, or from -0.50 to 5.0 D without astigmatism. The current approved hyperopia treatment range is from +1.50 to +4.0 D with less than 1.0 D of astigmatism.

There are some definite advantages to treating hyperopia with the Summit Apex Plus. The treatment zone is a full 6.5 mm and the Axicon lens is used to extend the transition zone out to 9.5 mm. The treatment zone portion of the procedure is performed with the iris diaphragm completely open and is delivered through the ablatable PMMA disc. There is no need to shield the hinge during the treatment zone portion of the procedure, which makes it easier to concentrate on maintaining perfect alignment over the pupil. The leading edge of the ablation can be seen on the stromal surface when performing the treatment zone. The most critical central laser pulses are delivered at the end of the ablation and are clearly visible. This ability to see the shape change over the central treatment zone helps to avoid decentered treatments. The hinge is then shielded when the Axicon lens is used (when performing the transition zone out to 9.5 mm).

Recent improvements have made this laser even easier to use. There is a new upgrade to the Apex Plus called the Infinity (Summit Technology, Inc, Waltham, Mass) package. Instead of having foot controls for movement of the patient chair, there is now a joystick control on the surgeon chair. During treatments, however, we recommend making small adjustments by manually moving the patient's head. There is some lag time in the electronic controls of any laser system chair. We believe that direct manual control of the patient is best for making micro adjustments to maintain perfect centration of the ablation. There is a new generation Zeiss microscope (Carl Zeiss Inc, Thornwood, NJ) with an electronic zoom that has improved the visualization for the surgeon. In addition to the standard HeNe beams, the Infinity upgrade also has a projected reticle to aid in centration.

Other important points to remember during these procedures involve the alignment system for treating astigmatism. It is important to make sure that the disc alignment template used in the preoperative laser testing is no longer in the Emphasis cassette (Summit Technology, Inc, Waltham, Mass). The toric erodable discs are then placed in the Emphasis cassette after making sure that it is aligned with the minus cylinder axis. Another way to check proper axis of the intended treatment is to tape a copy of the patient's topography to the laser. After the disc is properly aligned, make sure that there is no lint present on the disc surface before placing it into the down tube of the laser. If any lint is noted, it can easily be removed with compressed air.

In summary, the Summit Apex Plus is a good broadbeam laser that has recently been improved with the addition of the Infinity upgrade. It is capable of treating a wide range of refractive errors and has some features that make it especially effective in the treatment of hyperopia. Remembering a few key points when using the laser can help to avoid any problems when treating patients.

THE AUTONOMOUS LASER
(AUTONOMOUS TECHNOLOGIES CORPORATION, ORLANDO, FLA)
Marguerite B. McDonald, MD

Customized Corneal Ablations: The LASIK of the Future

Customized corneal ablations have captured the attention of all excimer laser surgeons. They hold the key to providing "super vision" for our patients (ie, better than 20/20 visual acuity). Customization has been the result of a gradual revolution via innovations such as wavefront sensors (Hartmann-Shack and Tscherning) and aberrocopes that can measure all of the eye's optical aberrations. Customized measurements allow us to deliver customized treatments.

The first customized corneal ablation in the world was performed in June 1999 by Theo Seiler, MD, using a 1.0 mm spot laser manufactured by Wavelight, Inc. (Erlangen, Germany) Two days postoperative, the patient's visual acuity improved from 20/12 best corrected to 20/10 uncorrected (presented at the International Society of Refractive Surgery Mid-Summer meeting, Miami, Florida, July 1999).

On October 12, 1999, Dr. Marguerite McDonald treated five patients with the CustomCornea hardware and software upgrade to the Autonomous laser, using a 0.8 mm flying spot. One eye of each patient was randomized to the ATC LADARVision (Autonomous Technologies Corporation, Orlando, Fla) traditional treatment, while the contralateral eye was treated with the customized treatment on a Hartmann-Shack type wavefront sensor called the CustomCornea measurement device (CCMD, Autonomous Technologies). On the first postoperative day, four of the five patients preferred the vision in the CustomCornea treated eye (presented at the annual meeting of International Society of Refractive Surgery, Orlando, Fla, October 1999, as well as the Refractive Surgery Interest Group Sub-Specialty Day meeting of the American Academy of Ophthalmology, Orlando, Fla, October 1999).

Within the past year, virtually every laser company has begun to approach customizing ablation based on wavefront aberration measurements. Corneal topography researchers have also started working with the laser companies to develop corneal ablations guided by corneal topography; yet other researchers are working on combined approaches that incorporate both wavefront and corneal topographic information.

There are actually three types of customized ablations. The first is functional customization based on patient's need, which has actually been in use for many years. The surgeon customizes the patient's treatment based on age, the presence or absence of presbyopia, occupational and recreational needs, refraction, and the psychological tolerance of the patient.

A second type of customization is anatomical, this type of customization has also been in widespread use for many years. The surgeon takes into consideration the corneal diameter and thickness, the pupil size, the anterior chamber depth, the anterior and posterior lens shape, and the axial length of each patient when designing the treatment pattern.

The third type of customization is optical; subtle aberrations in the wavefront are measured in this customization scheme. The customization can be based upon corneal topography and wavefront measurement (these include the Hartmann-Shack wavefront sensor, the Howland & Howland aberrometer, Tscherning's method, the Tracey system, slit light bundle approaches, and other new approaches as well).

The Autonomous CustomCornea program began, as stated above, on October 12, 1999, in New Orleans. This was the first time that aberration-free, wavefront-based customized ablations were attempted in the United States. Below are reported the results to date of the ATC investigational trial in the United States for customized LASIK ablations.

The FDA feasibility trial includes 20 patients who underwent bilateral LASIK and 20 patients undergoing bilateral PRK. One eye has been randomly selected for CustomCornea, and one eye has been selected for treatment with conventional LADARVision surgery. Myopic, hyperopic, and astigmatic corrections have all been included. We use the negative cylinder convention throughout our study, and "hyperopia" means positive sphere (ie, some "hyperopes" have negative spherical equivalent refractions preoperatively).

The right and left eyes must agree preoperatively to within 1 D in the spherical and cylindrical components, as must the wavefront/phoropter agreement preoperatively. The "match" parameter must have a value of greater than or equal to 0.5 (this indicates goodness of fit).

The LADARVision correction is always based on manifest phoropter refraction for myopic patients and cycloplegic refraction for hyperopic patients. The LADARVision cylinder is corrected if it is greater than or equal to 0.5 D. The optical zone for all patients is 6.5 mm in diameter (the wavefront data is available on greater than or equal to 7 mm in all cases). A blend zone of 1.25 mm is utilized in all CustomCornea patients as well as LADARVision patients receiving hyperopic and/or cylindrical correction.

Of the 20 LASIK patients treated, we have greater than or equal to 1 month follow-up data on 13 patients, with 1 week of data available on seven patients. The first three PRK patients were treated for myopia during the week prior to this wavefront meeting, therefore no data are yet available.

The initial five myopic LASIK patients treated on October 12, 1999, had between 2.00 and 3.75 D of myopia and up to -1.25 D of cylinder preoperatively. At 1 month postoperative, the uncorrected visual acuities (UCVAs) ranged between 20/16 and 20/25 in the CustomCornea eyes, and 20/12.5 to 20/25 in the conventional eyes. Three of the five patients saw better in their conventional eyes than they did in their CustomCornea eyes. One month BCVAs improved in both eyes of two patients.

It is important to note that visual acuity was always tested with a back-lit EDTRS chart in a 4 m exam lane, with room illumination at the patient's eye set at 12 to15 cd/m².

The assessment of myope group 1 was that the CustomCornea eyes appeared to be slightly overcorrected. An algorithm modification was made prior to treating myopic group 2 to account for this.

The remaining myopic LASIK patients were treated in November 1999 and January 2000 for a total of five additional patients, treated for up to 4 D of myopia and -1.75 D of astigmatism. This time, all five patients saw better in their CustomCornea eyes than their conventional eyes (CustomCornea UCVAs ranged from 20/12.5 to 20/20, and the conventional UCVAs ranged from 20/16 to 20/25).

Four out of five CustomCornea eyes had better BCVA postoperatively than they had preoperatively versus three out of five conventional eyes at 1 month postoperative.

This group of patients included one patient who had a postoperative decrease in her higher-order aberrations when compared to the preoperative value (0.15 microns RMS postoperatively, as compared to 0.22 microns preoperatively) in her CustomCornea eye; her conventional eye had a near doubling of the higher-order aberrations (0.25 microns RMS postoperatively, as compared to 0.14 microns preoperatively). This was the first time in the United States that a LASIK patient received an intentional and successful decrease in higher-order aberrations post-operatively when compared to preoperative values.

At 1 month postoperative, myope group 2 was assessed to have significantly improved outcomes in the CustomCornea eyes as the result of the algorithm modification that had been made, with all five CustomCornea eyes having better UCVAs than the five conventional eyes, and with BCVA improved over preoperative values in four of the five CustomCornea eyes (versus three out of five conventional eyes).

The initial three hyperopic LASIK patients were treated in December 1999 for between 2.0 and 3.0 D of hyperopia, and up to -1.75 D of astigmatism. At 1 month postoperative, all three conventional eyes had better UCVA than the CustomCornea eyes (though one eye had occult trauma just prior to the 1 month visit, resulting in a displaced flap with the presence of fresh blood noted at the slit lamp; the visual acuity measurements were taken prior to refloating of the flap. This patient had a UCVA of 20/25 1 month after the refloat.).

The 1 month postoperative BCVA of these three patients indicated that only one of the six eyes had better BCVA postoperatively as compared to preopera-tively, and this was a conventional eye.

The assessment of hyperope group 1 was that there was a general undercor-rection of the sphere in the CustomCornea eyes. It has been our conventional surgical experience that hyperopic patients require a 50% increase in the sphere term; an algorithm adjustment had been made for the conventional eyes but not for the CustomCornea eyes. The CustomCornea algorithm was therefore modi-fied to include this correction prior to the treatment of hyperope groups 2 and 3.

The remaining hyperopic patients were treated in January 2000, for a total of seven additional patients. They were treated for up to 4.25 D of hyperopia and up to -3.25 D of astigmatism. At 1 month postoperative, four of the seven patients saw better with their CustomCornea eyes versus three out of the seven who saw better with their conventional eyes. This postoperative data actually represents only 1 week of follow-up for six out of the seven patients. Postoperative BCVA was better than preoperative measurements for three of the seven CustomCornea eyes, as compared to one of the seven conventional eyes.

Hyperopic groups 2 and 3 were assessed to have improved clinical outcomes for the CustomCornea eyes based on the algorithm modification, with the CustomCornea UCVAs better than those for the conventional eyes in four of seven cases (based on 1 week data for six of the seven patients), and BCVA was improved over preoperative in three of seven CustomCornea eyes (versus one of seven conventional eyes). Though encouraged, the investigators feel there is still room for significant improvement.

When high-order aberrations are considered for the 12 patients with 1-month data, eight of the 12 patients (myopes and hyperopes) had smaller postoperative higher-order wavefront errors in the CustomCornea eyes than in the convention-al eyes. One patient out of 12 (a CustomCornea myope) had larger higher-order wavefront errors after surgery than before treatment; no conventional eyes showed this improvement.

The average higher-order RMS error for the CustomCornea eyes was 0.28 ±0.70 microns, and was 0.30 ±0.09 microns for the conventional eyes. No eyes lost more than one line BCVA in either group.

In summary, this stage feasibility trial has allowed us to treat patients, learn from them, and improve. The standardized testing conditions are essential, the investigators feel, to evaluate treatment efficacy, and the randomization of treatment for both eyes of each patient (ie, one eye CustomCornea, one eye conventional) is the ideal study design. Algorithm modifications have been identified and implemented at each stage, resulting in improved visual outcomes for the CustomCornea patients (particularly for the myopes). Additional work is needed to realize the full potential of the wavefront approach.

THE BAUSCH & LOMB TECHNOLAS 217C
Jaime R. Martiz, MD

The Bausch & Lomb Technolas 217 C laser has the latest PlanoScan ablation and flying spot technology on the market. It has a filtered air system that automatically cleans the optics each time the laser is switched on, reducing the need for maintenance and complications.

Complications directly related to the Technolas 217 may be serious but can largely be eliminated if the laser is in proper working order and energy level, beam centration, and beam quality are critically evaluated before each case. A malfunction of the laser could be due to dirty or damaged mirrors, defects in the laser optics, or inadequate gas (fluorine). It is important to understand that the laser is an ever-fluctuating instrument that is highly dependent on room temperature, barometric pressure, altitude, air purity, and humidity. Furthermore, the Bausch & Lomb service technicians must perform regular maintenance.

The following parameters correlate with complications that may result from not checking the Bausch & Lomb Technolas laser prior to ablation:

Parameters	*Complications*
Energy level	Poor ablation
Homogeneity of the beam	Uneven ablation
Optical system	Incorrect optic zone
Eye tracking system	Decentered ablation
Alignment beams	Overcorrection-undercorrection
Patient data inserted in the computer	

This laser is subject to a number of steps that must be followed in order to obtain an appropriate calibration. If the evaluation is not quantitative and qualitative, the surgeon could have a complication. The outcome of LASIK requires each pulse to have specific energy and homogeneity. If the surgeon does not check the emission from the laser at every operating session or between cases, the result could be undercorrection, because it varies from time to time and optics degrade.

The laser computer is programmed to deliver a specific number of pulses of a specific shape for each diopter to be corrected, and there is an internal monitoring system for fluence. However, an external check is always necessary. Fluence represents the quantity of energy the laser beam has when leaving the cavity, and it is 130 mJ/cm^2 for this particular laser. The total number of pulses necessary to obtain a complete exposure of the PMMA plate must equal 65 ±2, and any alterations in fluence can alter the cut rate in a direct proportional way. Poor fluence of the laser beam can result in poor photoablation. A satisfactory homogeneity of a 2.0 mm spot ensures that the same quantity of energy is delivered on all the points of its surface. In normal conditions, there is a color change from white to red (PMMA) in an interval of less than six spots. A very fine and diffuse white granularity can remain, but its elimination with a further spot can lead to a useless energy overload. Our experience taught us to perform a gas refill when, after increasing energy, we do not achieve a considerable reduction in the number of spots to obtain ablation.

The ablation surface can be altered by a small transition zone caused by a decentered or small hinge, fluid near the hinge or in other areas, or an inappropriate nomogram. During the ablation, fluid can accumulate on the corneal surface and should be wiped dry with a surgical spear (Merocel—Solan Ophthalmics, Jacksonville, Fla). It is important to cover the corneal hinge with a blunt instrument to prevent a double ablation. Usually ablation of the back surface of the corneal flap will result in induced irregular astigmatism. Uneven ablation surfaces produce decrease of visual acuity, reduction in contrast sensitivity, and alterations in quality of vision. It is important that the surgeon understands the reasons underlying these complications.

The Technolas 217 contains an active and passive eye tracker, derived from the most sophisticated military tracking systems, which compensates for eye micromovements without stopping the treatment. The tracking range is 1.5 mm. This means that during treatment a patient's eye movement exceeding 3.0 mm causes the ablation to stop. The treatment can start again from the point at which it was stopped when the patient resumes fixation and the eye-tracking system recognizes the memorized image. A high resolution infrared video camera and computer jointly track the eye. Initialization is a preliminary procedure before capturing by the eye tracker can begin. This is a step for the instrument to make an initial calibration in the gray range, depending on the color of the iris and diameter of the pupil. Therefore, the eye tracker should not be used in cases of ectopic pupil, infrared blurring, or coloboma of the iris. The two infrared light sources must be positioned at a 30° angle of inclination, with respect to the corneal bed and at a distance of 3.0 cm from the corneal apex. To avoid complication in this particular step, positioning of the infrared light source, focusing and centering must be perfectly performed shortly before lifting the flap because the ablation depends heavily on correctly performing this step.

Other complications are related to the patient's head positioning. The forehead and chin should be at the same level to result in a same amount of scleral show superiorly and inferiorly and that the corneal surface is perpendicular to the and assistant should verify proper laser setting.

Decentrations can be avoided by a preoperative check of laser centration. Ensure that the patient is always alert and continues to maintain fixation on the target point, and that centration is on the entrance pupil. Frequent monitoring of the beam position during the ablation by the surgeon should be performed. The patient should be reminded to stare at the target light. Sedation of patients should be reduced to a minimum or avoided completely.

If a significant decentration occurs, the best approach is to use Zioptix (Bausch & Lomb Surgical, Munich, Germany). This procedure is the combination or zylink of the abberrometer (wavefront measurement), Orbscan II (Orbtec, Inc, Salt Lake City, UT) and Technolas 217Z (Bausch & Lomb Surgical, Munich, Germany), which is an alternative being used by the Technolas 217 laser. The basic concept is to create a specific laser ablation treatment for correction of defects such as decentration, central islands, and irregular astigmatism. In this technique, the data acquired from the Orbscan topography system is copied and sent to Bausch & Lomb Surgical Technolas. Technolas calculates a session file, transfers the information by e-mail, and it is loaded into the Technolas 217 excimer laser just prior to treatment. The surgeon also receives a pictorial depicting the patient and treatment data, the preoperative corneal topographic map, the calculated ablation, and the predicted postoperative corneal topography map. By doing this, unwanted visual symptoms like glare or halos should be markedly decreased, if not eliminated.

LASER SCAN LSX (LASERSIGHT TECHNOLOGIES, INC, WINTER PARK, FLA)
*Technical information provided by Angela Q. King, MD,
Director of Education and Training, LaserSight Technologies, Inc*

The LaserScan LSX has FDA approval for PRK for the reduction or elimination of mild to moderate myopia (-1.0 to <-6.0 D) with ≤1.0 D astigmatism in patients with documentation of a stable manifest refraction (±0.5 D) over the past year and in patients who are 18 years or age or older. Approval of the application was based on a US study of 275 eyes with preoperative myopia <-6.0 D treated and followed for 6 months, with 181 of these eyes followed for 12 months or longer. In this study, 20/373 (5.4%) eyes were retreated. Of the 20 retreated eyes, seven eyes reached the 6 month follow-up visit for analysis. The physician may opt to treat up to -10.0 D.

Outcomes

The US study found that of the treated eyes, excluding data collected after retreatment, and based on refractive data at the ≥12 month follow-up examination, 85.37% were corrected to 20/40 or better without spectacles or contact lenses. For the retreated eyes that had reached the 6 month visit, 100% were corrected to 20/40 or better without spectacles or contact lenses. Adverse events at 12 months included: loss of one line or more of BCVA (1.1%), moderate corneal haze (1.2%), discomfort or pain (1.2%), increased IOP by 6 to 10 mmHg (1.9%), overcorrections by >1.0 D (4.9%), halos or starbursts (9.7%), night vision problems (1.1%), clarity changes day to day (9.1%), burning or gritty feeling (4.6%), and double vision or ghosting (2.6%).

Eye Tracker

The eye tracker uses pattern recognition to follow eye movement in both an active and passive mode. Infrared light is used for illumination. The tracker will track movement within a 3.0 mm range. If the eye moves outside this zone, the beam will be deflected and no energy will be delivered to the cornea. There is no dilation needed and no on-eye apparatus.

Fluence, Pulse, Frequency, Pulse Area

The fluence at the eye is 80 to 100 mJ/cm². The pulse frequency is 100 Hz in the US model and 200 Hz in the international version. The ablation area per pulse is 0.8 mm to 1.0 mm.

Treatment Zones

The treatment zones in the domestic version are fixed at 6.0 mm optical zone and 7.0 mm transitional zone for myopia 6.0 D or below. In myopia of more than 6.0 D, the optical zone size is 5.5 mm and the transitional zone is 6.5 mm. In hyperopia, the treatment zone is 6.5 mm to 8.5 mm. In the international model, the zone sizes are at the surgeon discretion and may go up to 10.0 mm.

Myopic/Hyperopic/Astigmatism Capabilities and Ablation Patterns

In the US model, myopia up to 10.0 D may be treated. A supplement has been filed with the FDA for approval of astigmatism. Clinical trials for higher range myopia, hyperopia, hyperopic astigmatism, and mixed astigmatism are currently underway. The international version can treat up to 20.0 D of myopia, 6.0 D of cylinder, and 8.0 D of hyperopia.

Special Features

The LSX treats astigmatism in a cross cylinder format. In addition, it produces a spherical ablation in astigmatic patients by treating a 6.0 mm optical zone in both the major and minor axis. This is in contrast to other lasers currently in use that treat only 4.5 mm in the minor axis and 5.5 mm in the major axis, producing an asymmetric ablation zone. This method does remove less tissue but has been postulated to increase the risk of qualitative decreases in vision.

Scanning technology is utilized in the international model with topographic link for treatment of decentered ablations and complex refractive errors. The LSX is also designed to be easily mobile and utilizes a standard 110 V power supply.

Upcoming Modifications

Several changes to the ergodynamics are underway, including repositioning of the joystick, improved dual control lighting, and an illuminated and binocular reticule.

CONCLUSION

The surgeon should be familiar with the ergonomics of the laser system from an operation standpoint and be aware of the availability of foot as well as console xyz control and positions of knobs and switches for magnification and lighting. The availability of slit, coaxial, and gooseneck lighting is very helpful for visualization of the pupil, inspection of the flap for wrinkles or folds, and for inspection of the interface for debris.

Again, attention to detail will allow the surgeon to operate comfortably and put the patient at ease by giving detailed instructions as to fixation and what to expect with regard to system noise. A patient who is at ease is less likely to move and will aid in obtaining the best possible results.

REFERENCES

1. Stein HA, Cheskes AT, Stein RM. Basics of excimer laser technology and history. In: Stein HA, Cheskes AT, Stein RM. *The Excimer: Fundamental and Clinical Use.* 2nd ed. Thorofare, NJ: SLACK Incorporated; 1997:4.

2. Edmison DR. Complications of photorefractive keratectomy. In: Freidlander MH, ed. *International Ophthalmology Clinics. Current Concepts of Refractive Surgery.* Philadelphia, Pa: Lippincott-Raven Publishers; 1997;37(1):83-94.

3. Slade SG. Abnormal induced topography. Central Islands. In, Machat JJ, ed. *Excimer Laser Refractive Surgery: Practice and Principles.* Thorofare, NJ: SLACK Incorporated; 1996:399.

4. Filatov V, Vidaurri-Leal JS, Talamo JH. Selected complications of radial keratotomy, photorefractive keratectomy, and laser in situ keratomileusis. In: Freidlander MH, ed. *International Ophthalmology Clinics. Current Concepts in Refractive Surgery.* Philadelphia, Pa: Lippincott-Raven Publishers, 1997;37(1):123-148.

5. O'Donnell CB, Kemner J, O'Donnell FE, Jr. Ablation smoothness as a function of excimer laser delivery system. *J Cataract Surg.* 1996;22(6):682-685.

4

LASIK Results: Safety, Efficacy, and Learning Curve

There has been extensive discussion of a definite learning curve for LASIK in the literature.[1-5] Slade reports that after having performed more than 2000 LASIK cases, the rate for minor complications such as irregular astigmatism is 1% to 2% and 0.2% to 0.3% for major complications (decreased from a total complication rate of 25% in the first 40 cases).[6] Tables 4-1 and 4-2 outline the safety of myopic LASIK as reported in the literature.[5,7-15] The series range in size from 21 cases to 1062 cases, and the percentage loss of two or more lines of BCVA ranges from 0% to 15.02%. Note in Table 4-2 that the degree of myopia correlates with the complication rate, and the highest complication rate is reported in a small series (32 eyes) of mean preoperative error 18.58 D. The loss of two or more lines of BCVA in our experience is less than 1%.

Results reported by Ditzen, et al for hyperopia up to 8.00 D indicated good predictability and stability up to 4.00 D.[16] Other studies indicate that the safety and efficacy of eyes treated for +4.25 to +8.00 D was good; however, there was regression and undercorrection in 12.9% of eyes at 6 months.[17] Epithelial ingrowth was reported to range from 15% to 31.4% in these studies. The incidence of epithelial ingrowth may be related to the use of a larger transition zone with spillover of the ablation over the edges of the bed. Because of this risk, the

Table 4-1

Safety and Efficacy of LASIK

Complication	Gimbel, et al[1] N = 1000		Stulting, et al[2] N = 1062	
	n	*%*	*n*	*%*
Gain of one or more lines BCVA	42	4.2	364	34.3
Gain of two or more lines BCVA	7	0.7	74	7.0
Loss of one or more lines BCVA	45	4.5	232	21.8
Loss of two or more lines BCVA	16	1.6	50	4.7
	N = 1000		*N = 1530**	
Shifted flap	12	1.2	13	0.85
Microwrinkles	11	1.1	2	0.13
Epithelial ingrowth	10	1.0	23	1.50

*These are reported over 1062 primary plus 468 enhancement procedures.

larger flap created by the Hansatome and other microkeratomes may be advantageous for hyperopic LASIK. In addition, LASIK appears to have a lower risk for haze and regression than hyperopic PRK. Zaldivar et al reported 576 hyperopic eyes treated with LASIK (average +3.88 hyperopic SE in one group and +4.68 SE with +2.55 D cylinder in a second group).[18] They reported 93% with an UCVA of >20/40 in group 1 and 60% with UCVA of >20/40 in group 2 postoperatively. They further reported a trend toward regression in the first 6 months postoperatively, which they felt was due to epithelial hyperplasia at the transition zone borders. Further investigations will be necessary to determine long-term stability and increase predictability of hyperopic LASIK.

The concept of the LASIK learning curve has received widespread attention.[1-5] Our experience confirms the presence of a learning curve in terms of the surgeon's facility with the microkeratome and with the recognition of anatomic features that may predispose to complications. We have reported intraoperative and postoperative complications and surgery times of the first 1000 myopic LASIK cases performed by one surgeon.[5] There were 19 microkeratome complications, 11 of which occurred in the first 226 cases. Only a single complication was reported in the final 200 cases in our series. There were no sight-threatening complications. The average keratometry in all uncomplicated cases was 44.24 D. This compared to average keratometry readings of 45.9 D in cases that resulted in thin flaps—46.7 D for buttonholes and 40.94 D for free caps.

The time between turning the flap and ablation as well as the total surgery time also decreased over the first 1000 cases, illustrating the learning curve of a single surgeon (Figures 4-1a and b). We also noted that the complication rates of a surgeon at our center who had begun performing LASIK at a later date were also decreased; this probably reflects the importance of mentoring and the sharing of experience between surgeons. Our most recent rates over 4015 cases are outlined in Tables 4-3a and b.

Table 4-2

LASIK Results

Study	Preoperative Refractive Error (D)	Number of Eyes	Postoperative Refractive Error (D)†	Duration of Follow-Up	Loss of Two or More Lines of BCVA
Gimbel, et al†	Mean −9.56 Range −1.00 to −23.00 20.00 −15.00 to −20.00 −10.00 to −14.99 <−10.00	8 55 319 618	(Overall results) 58.7%±0.50 83.4%±1.00 95.2%±2.00	Mean 3.8 months	1.7%
Thompson, et al†	Mean −7.20 D±3.10 (SD)	320	(Overall results) 62.1%±0.50 78.4%±1.00 95%±2.00	5.3±1.3 (SD) months	2.5%
Cauthier-Fournet†	Mean −4.46±0.51 (SD) Mean −7.51±1.90 (SD) Mean −12.46±1.48 (SD) Mean −18.58±3.20 (SD)	18 257 141 32	88.9%±1.0 100%±2.0 71.42%±1.0 96.01%±2.0 51.77%±1.0 82.9%±2.0 12.5%±1.0 71.88±2.0	3 months	0% 8.55% 9.21% 15.02%
Perez-Santonja, et al	Mean −13.19±2.89 (SD) Range −8.00 to −20.0	143	Mean +0.18±1.66	6 months	1.4%
Pallikaris	*Mean −11.53±1.77 (SD) Range −8.50 to −14.00	21	90.47%±2.00	1 year	0%
	Mean −18.14±3.04 Range −15.00 to −25.87	18	88.90%±2.00		0%
Tsai	Mean −5.44±1.36 Mean −8.41±0.84 Mean −12.65±1.51 Mean 19.53±2.61	29 26 40 19	Mean −0.02±0.50 Mean −0.37±1.04 Mean −0.62±1.23 Mean −0.65 ±2.99	9 months	0% 7.69% 5.00% 0%

Table 4-2 continued

LASIK Results

Study	Preoperative Refractive Error (D)	Number of Eyes	Postoperative Refractive Error (D)†	Duration of Follow-Up	Loss of Two or More Lines of BCVA
Pirzada, Kalaawry	Mean –2.09	85	UCVAΔ20/30 93%	Mean 48 days	<1% (1 eye)
Maldonado-Bas, Onis	–3.00 to –6.00	28	66.66%±1.00 33.33%±2.00	6 to 25 months	
	–6.25 to –10.00	138	63.00%±1.00 29.92%±2.00		3.14%
	–10.25 to –15.00	91	52.25%±1.00 35.71%±2.00		7.05%
	–15.25 to –25.50	43	32.50%±1.00 42.50%±2.00		2.50%
Waring, et al‡	–2.00 to –23.00 (mean –7.00)	995**	51.3%±0.50 77.8%±1.00	Follow-up 3 to 12 months	3.3%
Ojeimi, Waked	Mean +6.60 Range +3.00 to +10.25	21	Mean +220 Range –2.00 to +7.00	Mean 2.3 months	Not available
Ditzen, et al	Mean +2.50±1.70 Range +1.00 to +4.00	20	Mean +0.33±1.12	1 year	10%
	Mean +5.28±1.92 Range +4.25 to 8.00	23	Mean +1.91±1.83		4%

*An additional four eyes developed postoperative complications and were excluded from further analysis.
SD = 1 standard deviation
†Study results are expressed as percentage of eyes within emmetropia (eg, 58.7%±0.50 indicates that 58.7% of the eyes were within ±0.5 D of emmetropia).
**196 eyes also had Arc T for astigmatism.
‡Stulting RD, Balch K, Carr JD, Walter K, Thompson KP, Waring III GO. Complications of LASIK. *Invest Ophthalomol Vis Sci.* [ARVO Abstract] *1997;38(4):S231. Abstract # 1085.*
Adapted from Gimbel HV, Levy SG. LASIK: Results, indications, and complications. Current Opinion in Ophthalmology. 1998; 9(4).

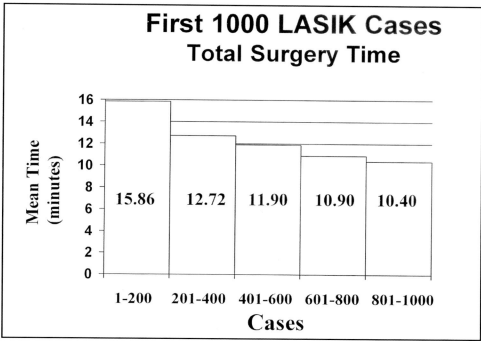

Figure 4-1a. There was a decrease in the total surgery time over the first 1000 LASIK cases performed by one surgeon at our center.

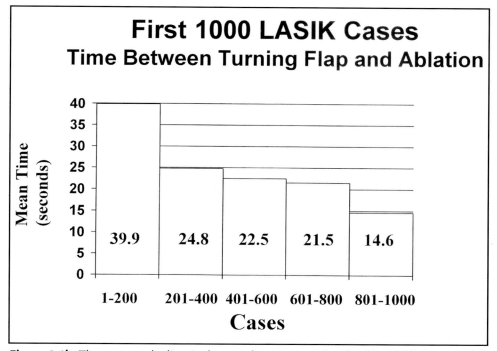

Figure 4-1b. There was a decline in the time between turning the flap and beginning the laser ablation over the same 1000 cases.

Table 4-3a		
Perioperative Flap Repositioning		
N = 4015		
	N	%
Shifted flap	33	0.82
Microwrinkles	8	0.20
Edge fold	5	0.12

(Reprinted with permission from Gimbel HV, Anderson Penno EE. LASIK Complications: Prevention and Management. Thorofare, NJ: SLACK Incorporated, 1999.)

Table 4-3b		
Microkeratome Complications and Surgical Events		
N = 4015		
	N	%
Incomplete pass	23	0.58
Thin flap	15	0.37
Buttonhole	7	0.17
Free cap	8	0.20
Insufficient suction	18	0.45
Flap shrinkage	3	0.08

(Reprinted with permission from Gimbel HV, Anderson Penno EE. LASIK Complications: Prevention and Management. Thorofare, NJ: SLACK Incorporated, 1999.)

To optimize the learning experience, we advocate carefully recording details of each surgery. This is facilitated by computerized medical records. By analyzing outcomes and carefully reviewing problems and complications in a process of continuous improvement, we have benefited from our experience with myopic LASIK—as there were only two complications in the first 226 hyperopic LASIK cases. These two complications were free caps in cases with average keratometry readings of 39.9 D and 42.0 D. As mentioned earlier, we have learned through our analysis of the first 1000 myopic LASIK cases that flat corneas may predispose to free caps.

A detailed discussion of LASIK complications with specific strategies to avoid them, as well as management of complications, will follow. It is essential to recognize that many of the complications and techniques are interrelated. For example, inadequate suction may result from inadequate exposure, and inadequate exposure may also lead to microkeratome pass problems. The keys to avoiding complications are meticulous attention to detail and an indepth understanding of LASIK techniques. A summary of techniques currently in use at our center will be provided following the discussion of complications.

It is important to emphasize that despite extensive experience, complications can occur even when a skilled, experienced surgeon is operating. The surgeon must be aware of particular anatomic features that may predispose to complications. Mechanical failures may also lead to complications, but this can be minimized by careful maintenance, cleaning, assembly, and routine checks of equipment. Furthermore, a philosophy of continuous improvement means that important lessons may be learned from the first case as well as from the 3000th case.

REFERENCES

1. Gimbel HV, Basti S, Kaye GB, Ferensowicz M. Experience during the learning curve of laser in situ keratomileusis. *J Cataract Refract Surg.* 1996;22:542-550.

2. Perez-Santonja JJ, Bellot J, Claramonte P, Ismail MM, Alio JL. Laser in situ keratomileusis to correct high myopia. *J Cataract Refract Surg.* 1997;23:372-385.

3. Marinho A, Pinto C, Pinto R, Vaz F, Castro Neves M. LASIK for high myopia: One year experience. *Ophthalmic Surg Lasers (Suppl).* 1996;27(5):S517-S520.

4. Handzel A. How to shorten the learning curve. In: Pallikaris IG, Siganos DS, eds. *LASIK.* Thorofare, NJ: SLACK Incorporated; 1998:153-163.

5. Gimbel HV, Anderson Penno EE, van Westenbrugge JA, Ferensowicz M, Furlong MT. Incidence and management of intra and early postoperative complications in 1000 consecutive LASIK cases. *Ophthalmology.* 1998;105:1839-1848

6. Slade SG. LASIK complications and their management. In: Machat JJ, ed. *Excimer Laser Refractive Surgery: Practice and Principles.* Thorofare, NJ: SLACK Incorporated; 1996:359.

7. Thompson KP, Carr JD, Warring III GO, Stulting RD. LASIK: The preliminary American experience. In: Pallikaris IG, Siganos D, eds. *LASIK.* Thorofare, NJ: SLACK Incorporated; 1998:223-231.

8. Gauathier-Fournet L. LASIK results. In: Pallikaris IG, Siganos D, eds. *LASIK.* Thorofare NJ: SLACK Incorporated; 1998:233-245.

9. Perez-Santonja JJ, Bellot J, Claramonte P, Ismail MM, Alio JL. Laser in situ keratomileusis to correct high myopia. *J Cataract Refract Surg.* 1997;23(3):372-385.

10. Pallikaris IG, Siganos DS. Laser in situ keratomileusis to treat myopia: Early experience. *J Cataract Refract Surg.* 1997;23(1):39-49.

11. Tsai RJ. Laser in situ keratomileusis for myopia of -2 to -25 diopters. *J Refract Surg.* 1997;13 (suppl):S427-429.

12. Pirzada WA, Kalaawry H. Laser in situ keratomileusis for myopia of -1 to -3.50 diopters. *J Refract Surg.* 1997;13 (suppl):S425-426.

13. Maldonado-Bas A, Onis R. Results of laser in situ keratomileusis in different degrees of myopia. *Ophthalmology.* 1998;105(4):606-611.

14. Ojeimi G, Waked N. Laser in situ keratomileusis for hyperopia. *J Refract Surg.* 1997;13 (suppl):S432-433.

15. Ditzen K, Huschka H, Pieger S. LASIK for hyperopia. In: Buratto L, Brint SF, eds. *LASIK: Principles and Techniques.* Thorofare NJ: SLACK Incorporated; 1998:269-275.

16. Ditzen K, Huschka H, Pieger S. Laser in situ keratomileusis for hyperopia. *J Cataract Refract Surg.* 1998;24(1):42-47.

17. Göker S, Er H, Kahvecioglu C. Laser in situ keratomileusis to correct hyperopia from +4.25 to +8.00 diopters. *J Refract Surg.* 1998;14(1):26-30.

18. Zaldivar R, Oscherow S, Ricur G. LASIK and Hyperopia. (Abstract #8). In: *American Society of Cataract and Refractive Surgery. Symposium on Cataract, IOL, and Refractive Surgery.* 1998:2.

5

Intraoperative Complications

Attention to detail on preoperative assessment as outlined in Table 2-2 may allow the surgeon to anticipate potential complications, counsel patients accordingly, and/or devise preoperative strategies.

INADEQUATE EXPOSURE

Inadequate exposure can lead to difficulties placing the suction ring, failure to achieve suction, and incomplete microkeratome passes (Table 5-1). Exposure is of particular concern when operating on the right eye with the ACS, because the stopper is located superiorly when operating on the right eye. It may catch on the upper lid or drapes, resulting in an incomplete pass.

Findings on the preoperative workup may forewarn of possible problems with inadequate exposure. For example, deep-set eyes, previous trauma such as orbital fractures, and/or narrow palpebral fissures should be noted prior to surgery. Inadequate palpebral fissure may require a lateral canthotomy (see Patient Example 4). Although, with careful draping and proper patient positioning, lateral canthotomy should rarely be necessary. In addition, poor draping techniques may result in inadequate exposure; if the drape is allowed to stick to itself, a

Table 5-1	
Inadequate Exposure	
Possible Causes	• Orbital anatomy (deep-set eyes, small palpebral fissure) • Prior orbital or lid trauma or surgery • Poor draping technique • Poor choice of lid speculum
Results	• Difficulty placing suction ring • Failure to achieve adequate suction • Incomplete microkeratome pass (interference from speculum and drape)
Solutions	*Prevention* • Careful draping techniques to maximize exposure • Strong spring or locking speculum • Chin-up or down head position to achieve central eye position • Assistant to provide downward pressure on speculum during microkeratome pass *Management* • Lateral canthotomy may be necessary in rare circumstances

pseudopalpebral fissure can be created that may be smaller than the actual palpebral fissure.

For maximum exposure, the drape should be held taut until it adheres to the lids. Manual separation of the lids with eversion of the lid margins and lashes while the drape is being applied will improve exposure and keep cilia out of the operative field (Figures 5-1a through e). It is helpful to have the scrub nurse assist with draping.

In addition, a speculum with a posteriorly angulated hinge will eliminate interference from the speculum when the microkeratome is placed (Figure 5-2). The lids may be held apart more effectively with a strong spring or locking speculum. As noted previously, patient head position can also affect exposure, and the patient should be positioned so as to maximize globe exposure. A slight chin-up position may be helpful, particularly in patients with prominent brows. We have learned that it is helpful to have the scrub or circulating nurse press down gently on the speculum while engaging the microkeratome; this moves the eyelids away from the path of the microkeratome and reduces conjunctival folds and redundancy where the suction ring contacts the globe and also proptoses the globe slightly to help avoid incomplete passes due to interference from the lid or drapes (Figure 5-3). When using the Hansatome, it is necessary to keep the lower eyelid away from the blade.

A lateral canthotomy can be performed if the lids cannot be separated enough to place the suction ring. However, with attention to detail when draping and positioning combined with the assistance with the speculum as described above, lateral canthotomy should be needed only in rare circumstances.

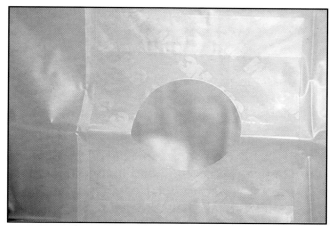

Figure 5-1a. Proper draping technique. A standard is cut. (Reprinted with permission from Gimbel HV, Anderson Penno EE. *LASIK Complications: Prevention and Management.* Thorofare, NJ: SLACK Incorporated, 1999.)

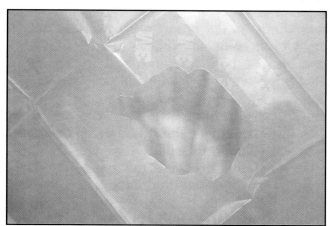

Figure 5-1b. A standard is cut, as demonstrated in Figure 5-1a, to aid in draping. (Reprinted with permission from Gimbel HV, Anderson Penno EE. *LASIK Complications: Prevention and Management.* Thorofare, NJ: SLACK Incorporated, 1999.)

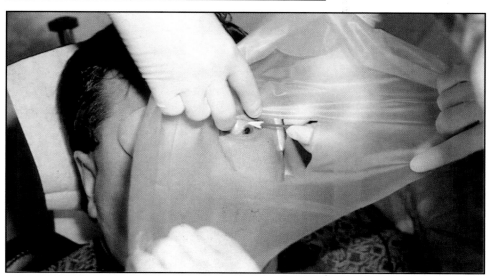

Figure 5-1c. The surgeon and assistant hold the drape taut while a sponge is used to evert the cilia of the upper lid. (Reprinted with permission from Gimbel HV, Anderson Penno EE. *LASIK Complications: Prevention and Management.* Thorofare, NJ: SLACK Incorporated, 1999.)

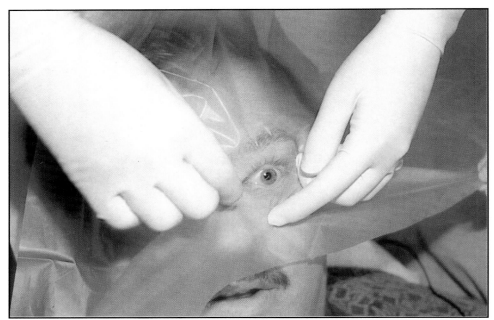

Figure 5-1d. The lower lid is similarly everted, and the speculum is placed. (Reprinted with permission from Gimbel HV, Anderson Penno EE. *LASIK Complications: Prevention and Management.* Thorofare, NJ: SLACK Incorporated, 1999.)

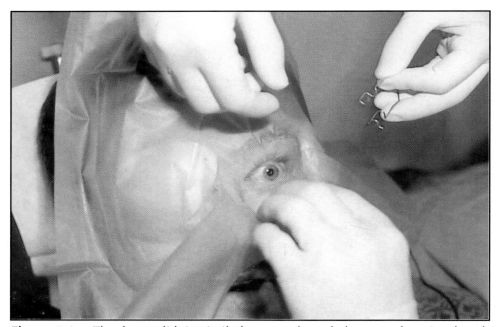

Figure 5-1e. The lower lid is similarly everted, and the speculum is placed. (Reprinted with permission from Gimbel HV, Anderson Penno EE. *LASIK Complications: Prevention and Management.* Thorofare, NJ: SLACK Incorporated, 1999.)

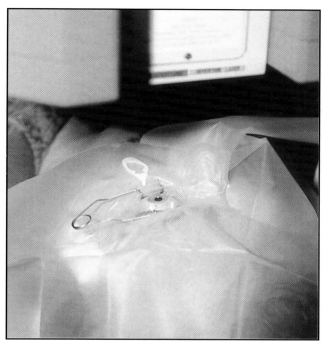

Figure 5-2. Lid speculum. A speculum with a posterior angulated hinge with a strong spring or locking mechanism should be used to optimize exposure. (Reprinted with permission from Gimbel HV, Anderson Penno EE. *LASIK Complications: Prevention and Management.* Thorofare, NJ: SLACK Incorporated, 1999.)

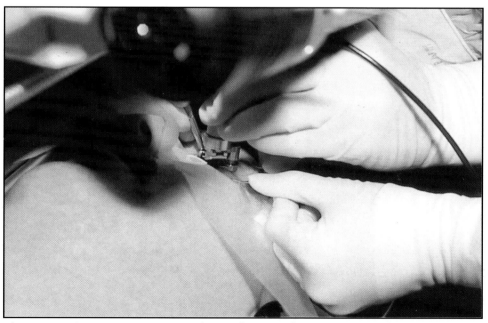

Figure 5-3. Optimizing exposure during the microkeratome pass. The assistant provides gentle downward pressure on the lid speculum as the microkeratome is passed to proptose the globe slightly and enhance exposure. (Reprinted with permission from Gimbel HV, Anderson Penno EE. *LASIK Complications: Prevention and Management.* Thorofare, NJ: SLACK Incorporated, 1999.)

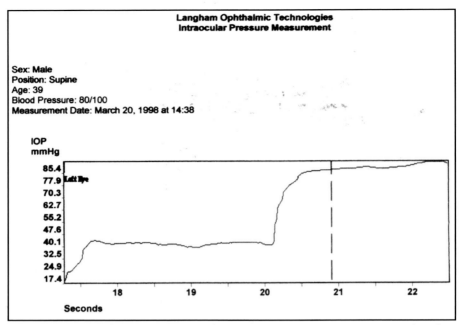

Figure 5-4a. Langham tonometry. The two-step rise in IOP is measured with a Langham tonometer as suction is applied just prior to performing the micro-keratome pass. (Reprinted with permission from Gimbel HV, Anderson Penno EE. *LASIK Complications: Prevention and Management.* Thorofare, NJ: SLACK Incorporated, 1999.)

INADEQUATE SUCTION

An optimal cut by the microkeratome depends on an IOP greater than 65 mmHg. IOPs of less than this may result in thin flaps or buttonholes (see Patient Example 4, 5, and 6). It is clear from preliminary studies that we have performed with the Langham tonometer (Orb Diagnostics, Brooklandville, Md) that there is a great variation in the IOP obtained and maintained after suction is applied and that the fluctuations in IOP are much more complex than is captured by simple Barraquer tonometry (Figures 5-4a and b) (Poster presentation at 1998 Annual Meeting. AAO, New Orleans. Variability of intraocular pressure after ring application in LASIK procedures research.) Further investigations will help to describe what is happening just before the microkeratome pass (with respect to IOP) and may help to correlate differences in IOP with the potential for flap complications.

To achieve the proper IOP, the suction ring must be properly placed and the suction port must be completely free from obstruction. Inadequate exposure is a common cause of inability to seat the suction ring, so care should always be taken when draping and positioning the patient prior to placement of the suction ring (Table 5-2). The suction ring should be held firmly against the globe until it is well seated. In cases where the corneal diameter is smaller than average, the suction ring will extend further beyond the limbus, allowing loose conjunctiva to tent and block the suction port if it is not held firmly against the globe.

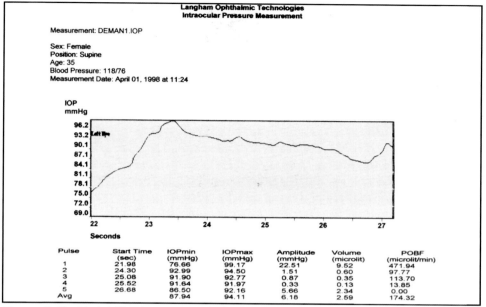

Figure 5-4b. Variability is measured after maximum suction is attained. (Reprinted with permission from Gimbel HV, Anderson Penno EE. *LASIK Complications: Prevention and Management.* Thorofare, NJ: SLACK Incorporated, 1999.)

Table 5-2

Inadequate Suction

Possible Causes	• Inadequate exposure • Small corneal diameter resulting in conjunctival tenting and blockage of the suction port • Manipulations of suction ring, drape, or speculum leading to loss of suction
Results	• Thin flap • Buttonhole
Solutions	*Prevention* • Attention to techniques that optimize exposure (see Table 5-1) • Hold suction ring firmly against globe so it is well-seated when turning suction on • Avoid manipulations of the suction ring and drapes or speculum • Always measure IOP with Barraquer tonometer or develop tactile sense of high IOP • Do not rely on the suction gauge, remeasure IOP if any manipulation is made *Management* • Release suction, re-adust head position, drapes, and speculum, and reposition suction ring • If successful with readjustments, use a smaller suction ring if available and if appropriate (hyperopic treatments may require a larger suction ring)

Figure 5-5. Barraquer tonometer. (Reprinted with permission from Gimbel HV, Anderson Penno EE. *LASIK Complications: Prevention and Management.* Thorofare, NJ: SLACK Incorporated, 1999.)

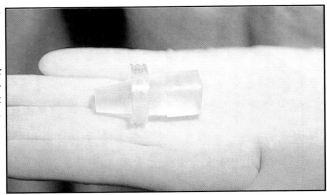

When placing the suction ring, firm pressure should be applied prior to turning on the vacuum. After the ring is seated, this pressure is then released to allow the eye to again proptose out of the orbit so that the microkeratome will clear the eyelids, drape, and speculum. Bear in mind that conjunctiva blocking the port can give a high reading on the gauge but no suction on the globe, to obtain an IOP of less than 65 mmHg. The IOP should always be measured with the Barraquer tonometer or other means and not assumed to be high simply because the vacuum limit on the pump has been reached (Figure 5-5). In addition, to avoid loss of suction, the suction ring should not be tilted or moved to any great extent. If any manipulations of the speculum, drapes, or lids are made, the IOP should be remeasured with the tonometer before the microkeratome pass.

In cases with difficulty placing the suction ring or inadequate suction, adjustments to the speculum and drapes will usually allow adequate suction on a second attempt. Generally, no more than three attempts can be made due to the swelling of the conjunctiva. In rare cases, LASIK may need to be postponed or a conversion made to PRK if appropriate.

MICROKERATOME COMPLICATIONS

Thin Flaps and Buttonholes

Thin flaps and buttonholes may be the consequence of inadequate suction. However, these complications can occur despite IOP greater than 65 mmHg (Figure 5-6).

In these cases, it may be corneal anatomy. Corneas that are steeper than average may be prone to buckling as excess tissue is compressed beyond plantation by the

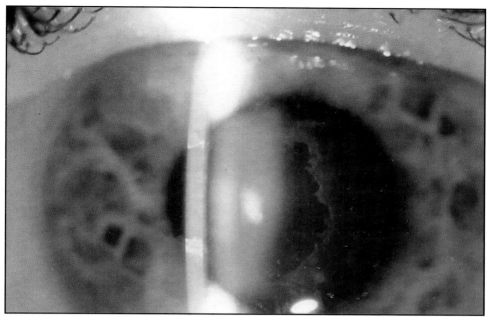

Figure 5-6. Buttonhole. This figure demonstrates retroillumination of a buttonhole obtained in Patient Example 4. (Reprinted with permission from Gimbel HV, Anderson Penno EE. *LASIK Complications: Prevention and Management.* Thorofare, NJ: SLACK Incorporated, 1999.)

foot plate of the microkeratome (see Patient Example 5). The microkeratome may make a complete pass, but the resulting flap will have central thinning or a buttonhole. The surgeon may also choose to counsel patients with corneal curvatures out of the normal range (<41.00 D and >46.00 D) that they may be at increased risk for flap complications (Figure 5-7).

Providing gentle upward support to the microkeratome handle when using the ACS may also help to avoid buttonholes that can result from torquing the microkeratome-suction ring assembly by the weight of the handle. Poor blade quality or microkeratome malfunctions may also predispose to these flap complications.[1] Poor blade quality can lead to irregular cuts with thin areas. Finally, the cut should be made continuously—without stopping and restarting midway through the microkeratome pass.

In most cases, adequate suction can be attained with proper draping and adequate exposure. One can avoid creating thin flaps and buttonholes due to inadequate IOP by appropriate measurements with the Barraquer tonometer after placement of the suction ring and after any adjustments; the case should be halted if IOP of 65 mmHg or more is not attained. The surgeon also may ask the patient to verify that the vision has dimmed significantly or blacked out, confirming high IOP and restriction of blood flow to the eye.

Avoiding flap complications due to equipment malfunction can be minimized by fastidious cleaning, assembly, and checking of the microkeratome prior to use. Cleaning basin water, ultrasonic cleaning water, and rinse water should be

Figure 5-7. Buttonhole/ thin flap. Steep (>45.00 D average keratometry reading) corneas are at risk for buttonhole or central thinning due to buckling of the cornea during the microkeratome pass. (Reprinted with permission from Gimbel HV, Anderson Penno EE. *LASIK Com=plications: Prevention and Management.* Thorofare, NJ: SLACK Incorporated, 1999.)

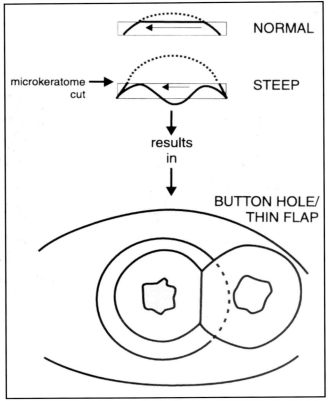

changed frequently. It is a standard of care to use a new blade for each patient in North America. In cases with steep corneas that do not require a high correction, choosing to make a 180 μ cut rather than a 160 μ cut may help avoid the risk of thin flaps or buttonholes. A different suction ring design, as well as a different footplate, may also help avoid these complications.

In a case where a buttonhole is created, the procedure should be stopped after replacing the flap and LASIK rescheduled at a later date. When recutting a flap after a buttonhole, a thicker plate (180 μ) should ideally be used. In the case of a thin flap without a buttonhole, but with faint ridges on the bed, an alternative is to proceed with the ablation. This should not be done, however, if the thin area is directly in the visual axis. One should be prepared to make the decision whether or not to proceed quickly to avoid desiccation of the flap and stromal bed. These points are summarized in Table 5-3.

Free Cap

Free caps may be the result of mechanical failure or anatomic features (Table 5-4). When using the ACS, the stopper should be advanced appropriately to avoid creating a free cap. The correct amount is determined by checking the blade travel in the microkeratome suction ring after assembly and before the cut. In our experience, despite proper microkeratome assembly, free caps have occurred in

Table 5-3

Thin Flaps and Buttonholes

Possible Causes
- Inadequate suction
- Corneal anatomy—excessively steep, irregular (eg, previous PKP), or high astigmatism
- Torque induced by the weight of the microkeratome assembly
- Poor blade quality

Results
- Inability to perform laser ablation
- Risk of epithelial ingrowth
- Risk of irregular astigmatism
- If LASIK performed at a later date, the flap will have to be recut

Solutions
Prevention
- Do not make the microkeratome pass if adequate IOP not verified
- Advise patients with unusually high or low keratometry readings of increased risk
- Consider using deeper depth plate on steep corneas
- Provide gentle upward support on the microkeratome handle during the pass (ACS)
- Use firm downward pressure on the suction ring during the pass (Hansatome)
- Check the microkeratome prior to each use
- It is standard care to use a new blade for each patient

Management
- Replace the thin flap or buttonholed flap while carefully managing the epithelial edges
- Inspect the flap meticulously and verify adherence
- Laser ablation may not be done in a case of a thin flap with ridges on the bed or with only a very thin cut of stroma
- Recut the flap with a thicker depth plate at a later date (2 to 3 months later)

Table 5-4	
Free Cap	
Possible Causes	• Failure to advance the stopper sufficiently on the corneal shaper • Corneal anatomy is large and flat (<41.00 mean keratometry) • Loss of suction during pass
Results	• Free cap • Ablation can proceed if complete free cap
Solutions	*Prevention* • Carefully check the entire microkeratome assembly, including the stopper, prior to each case • Corneal marks should be asymmetric to aid in proper cap replacement • Warn patients with large, flat corneas of the increased risk *Management* • Place the free cap in an antidesiccation chamber or keep it covered in the microkeratome while the ablation is done • Carefully replace the cap stromal side down with attention to orientation as aided by preoperative corneal marks • Assure adherence by waiting 3 to 5 minutes after cap replacement • Sutures are not necessary in most cases

large flat corneas of less than 41.00 D mean keratometry when using the ACS. This may have been due to the interaction of the microkeratome and suction ring with the globe.[1] A smaller area of the cornea may have been presented to the microkeratome blade, with these cases resulting in a free cap. One might think that eyes with smaller than average corneal diameters may have a higher risk of free cap, but this is not necessarily true. In these eyes, a larger percentage of the cornea is presented to the microkeratome blade due to the fact that the suction ring is seated on the surrounding limbus.[1]

Patients with flat corneas should be informed of the possible increased risk of flap complications. If a free cap is encountered, the cap should be kept covered in the microkeratome or carefully placed in an anti-desiccation chamber while ablation is performed. It is imperative to replace the cap stromal surface down. Careful corneal marking preoperatively is essential in proper replacement of a free cap. Some surgeons advocate the routine use of double circle markings with different sized circles to aid in the alignment if a free cap occurs. Alternatively, three asymmetrical linear marks may be made (Figure 5-8). After replacing the cap, place a few drops of balanced salt solution under the flap while holding it with a forceps and carefully remove fluid in the usual manner after the cap is aligned properly. Wait 3 to 5 minutes to ensure adherence of the free cap to the bed. It is not necessary to suture the cap in place. However, if disruption of the epithelium has occurred, a bandage contact lens may be placed (see Patient Example 7).

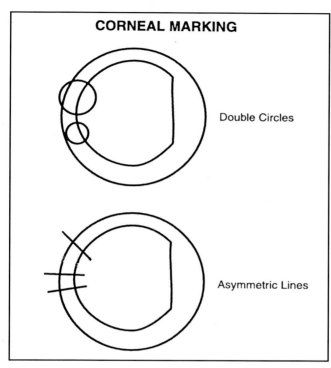

CORNEAL MARKING

Double Circles

Asymmetric Lines

Figure 5-8. Corneal marking. Corneal marking should be done with circles of different sizes or asymmetric lines such that in the event of a free cap, the cornea can be aligned properly. (Reprinted with permission from Gimbel HV, Anderson Penno EE. *LASIK Complications: Prevention and Management.* Thorofare, NJ: SLACK Incorporated, 1999.)

Incomplete Pass

Incomplete passes may be due to a variety of underlying causes (Table 5-5) (see Patient Example 10). A common cause of incomplete passes is interference from the lids, speculum, or drapes. As mentioned previously, this is of particular concern when operating on the right eye with the ACS. Debris or conjunctiva on the suction ring tracks, microkeratome gear, or obstruction by the drapes or eyelids may also lead to failure of the microkeratome to complete the pass. Another cause of microkeratome failure is improper assembly or cleaning, and more than tolerable friction in the pass of the microkeratome through the suction ring slots.

Complete knowledge of the microkeratome system is critical in these cases. A stop-start is inadvisable with the ACS; however, with the Hansatome, repeat steps on the forward pedal may generate enough power to overcome resistance and complete the pass. In the event of a partial pass with jamming of the microkeratome such that it cannot be reversed, the suction should be released and the microkeratome-suction assembly slid out gently away from the hinge. When a partial pass occurs, the surgeon must make the decision as to whether or not the ablation can proceed. If near the edge of the planned ablation, the hinge can be protected with a moist sponge (Figure 5-9). If the pass stops close to the pupil and certainly if it stops within the central 5 mm, the ablation cannot be performed and the flap should be repositioned. A LASIK recut can be performed after a 3-month wait. The surgeon should plan to recut the flap with a same depth plate. If it is felt that the incomplete pass was due to anatomic reasons, such as a narrow palpebral fissure, one should consider the need for lateral canthotomy.

Table 5-5

Incomplete Pass

Possible Causes	• Poor exposure—obstruction by drapes, lid, or speculum • Debris or conjunctiva on suction ring tracks • Improper assembly or cleaning of the microkeratome
Results	• Inability to proceed with the ablation if the pass stops within the central 6 to 7 mm zone
Solutions	*Prevention* • Use proper techniques to ensure adequate exposure (see Table 5-1), including lateral canthotomy in rare cases • Careful assembly, cleaning, and inspection of microkeratome and suction ring prior to each use • Run the microkeratome through a complete forward and reverse cycle prior to each eye to ensure proper functioning • Avoid excess fluid prior to microkeratome use, as BSS crystals may lead to motor head dysfunction in subsequent cases • Restart forward movement with the Hansatome. Never reverse and forward or stop-and-start with the ACS *Management* • If proceeding with laser ablation, shield the hinge with a sponge • If unable to perform ablation (if the pass stops within the central 5 mm), replace the flap and recut at a later date with the same depth plate

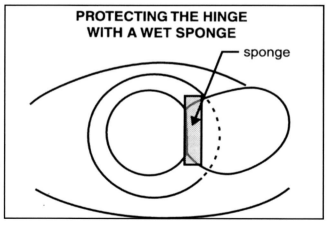

Figure 5-9. Hinge protection. In the event of a partial pass or a small corneal flap, the hinge should be protected with a moist sponge to avoid ablation of the flap and the hinge area, which may be a risk for epithelial growth. (Reprinted with permission from Gimbel HV, Anderson Penno EE. *LASIK Complications: Prevention and Management.* Thorofare, NJ: SLACK Incorporated, 1999.)

Prior to each surgery, the microkeratome and suction ring assembly should be inspected carefully under the operating microscope (see Table 3-1). Each microkeratome has features that are unique. The surgeon, as well as the scrub nurses, should be thoroughly familiar with the proper cleaning, assembly, and use of the particular microkeratome. The microkeratome should also be placed onto the suction ring and run through a complete forward and reverse pass cycle to ensure that it is functioning properly with no intolerable resistance prior to placing it on the eye. Balanced salt solution (BSS) crystals from previous surgeries not removed from the motor shaft can cause the motor head to malfunction; therefore, excess fluid should not be used in the operative field before the microkeratome pass, and any moisture on the shaft of the motor at the end of the surgery when the micro-keratome is disassembled should be immediately wiped off with a Merocel sponge. Using salt-free solutions (such as topical anesthetic rather than BSS) to moisten the cornea before the cut avoids these potential problems.

Corneal Perforation

Corneal perforation is a rare but devastating complication. It has been described with improper microkeratome assembly—specifically failure to place the depth plate into the ACS microkeratome head (Figures 5-10a through c). Improperly seat-ing the depth plate may also lead to a deeper cut and perforation. For this reason, the number of personnel handling the microkeratome should be limited, and the surgeon should always check the microkeratome carefully prior to use (Table 5-6).

Management of corneal perforation will depend on the depth of the cut. Cases in which the depth plate has been left out entirely have resulted in injury to the cornea, iris, and lens, and have necessitated corneal transplant and IOL implantation. Cases in which the depth plate is present but improperly seated will result in corneal perforation and iris injuries, but may not damage the lens. During the pre-operative informed consent process, it is necessary to warn patients that while LASIK is generally safe and effective, there is the unlikely possibility of sight-threatening complications.

FLAP COMPLICATIONS

Shifted Flap

Intraoperatively, shifted flaps may occur from unexpected eye movement when a sponge or instrument is close to the limbus but are most likely to occur as the speculum and drapes are being removed (Figures 5-11a and b). This can result from the patient squeezing the lids, causing a Bell's phenomenon when the specu-lum is lifted away. As a consequence, the eye turns up, and the flap is more likely to be dislodged by the drape or speculum.

To avoid this complication, we currently instruct the patients to continue looking straight ahead and not to squeeze their eyes as the speculum and drapes are taken away (Table 5-7). As an added precaution, we also hold the lids open with the thumb and forefinger during this maneuver (Figure 5-12). Should the flap become dislodged, the flap can be repositioned by refloating it, as described in Chapter 6. It is unlikely that folds or wrinkles will develop when the flap becomes dislocated intraoperatively and is repositioned immediately.

Wrinkled Flap

To avoid epithelial wrinkles, the flap should be positioned carefully as it is ini-tially turned for the ablation. The flap should lay as a cup (Figure 5-13). In addi-tion, excessive drying of the flap during the ablation may contribute to wrinkling. We recommend that the flap be placed on a damp sponge during the ablation.

Figure 5-10a. The 180-µm spacer is not fully inserted (compare to Figure 5-10b). (Reprinted with permission from Gimbel HV, Anderson Penno EE. *LASIK Complications: Prevention and Management.* Thorofare, NJ: SLACK Incorporated, 1999.)

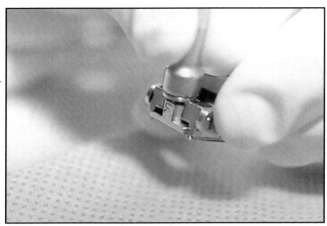

Figure 5-10b. The spacer ends are flush with the microkeratome assembly. (Reprinted with permission from Gimbel HV, Anderson Penno EE. *LASIK Complications: Prevention and Management.* Thorofare, NJ: SLACK Incorporated, 1999.)

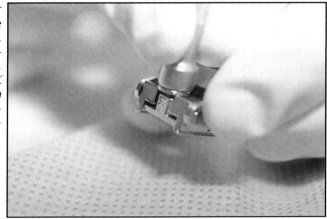

Figure 5-10c. To ensure proper placement, it may be helpful to hold the spacer in proper position while tightening it into place. (Reprinted with permission from Gimbel HV, Anderson Penno EE. *LASIK Complications: Prevention and Management.* Thorofare, NJ: SLACK Incorporated, 1999.)

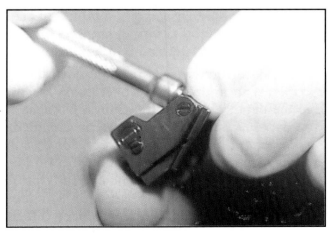

Table 5-6
Corneal Perforation

Possible Causes	• Failure to place the depth plate into the microkeratome assembly • Improperly seating the depth plate
Solutions	*Prevention* • Meticulous assembly and inspection of the microkeratome prior to each use *Management* • Dependent upon the depth of the cut • Corneal transplantation and IOL implantation may be needed in severe cases

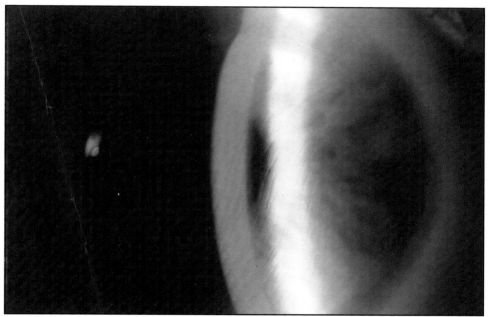

Figure 5-11a. This demonstrates a shifted flap before repositioning (see Patient Example 19). (Reprinted with permission from Gimbel HV, Anderson Penno EE. *LASIK Complications: Prevention and Management.* Thorofare, NJ: SLACK Incorporated, 1999.)

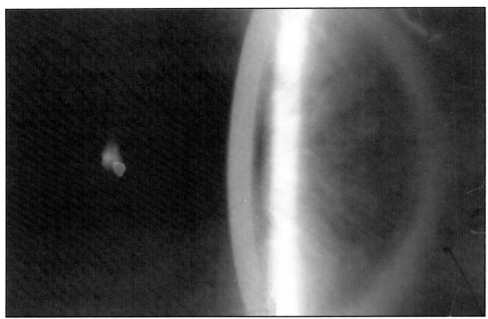

Figure 5-11b. This demonstrates a shifted flap after repositioning (see Patient Example 19). (Reprinted with permission from Gimbel HV, Anderson Penno EE. *LASIK Complications: Prevention and Management.* Thorofare, NJ: SLACK Incorporated, 1999.)

Table 5-7

Shifted Flap Intraoperatively

Possible Causes	• Movement of the eye when doing the striae test • Patient squeezing eyes as drapes and speculum are being removed
Results	• Flap dislocation or wrinkling
Solutions	*Prevention* • Have patient concentrate on the light when doing the striae test • Ask the patient to avoid squeezing and to look straight ahead as drapes and speculum are being removed • Hold the lids open with thumb and forefinger as the drapes and speculum are being removed *Management* • Immediately refloat the flap into position

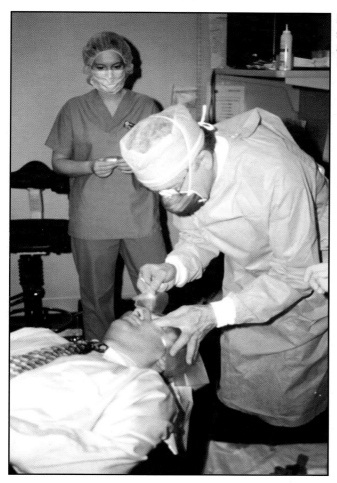

Figure 5-12. The lids are stabilized with the thumb and forefinger as the drape is removed.

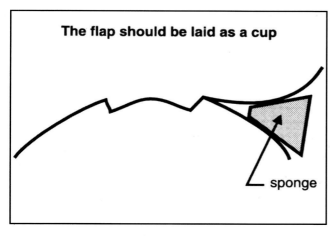

The flap should be laid as a cup

sponge

Figure 5-13. To avoid epithelial wrinkles, the flap should be laid as a cup as it is initially turned. This will help prevent wrinkles from forming during the ablation and aid in proper flap repositioning. (Reprinted with permission from Gimbel HV, Anderson Penno EE. *LASIK Complications: Prevention and Management.* Thorofare, NJ: SLACK Incorporated, 1999.)

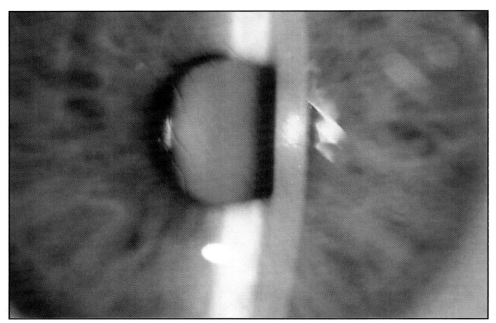

Figure 5-14. This is an example of wrinkles that are centrally located. (Reprinted with permission from Gimbel HV, Anderson Penno EE. *LASIK Complications: Prevention and Management.* Thorofare, NJ: SLACK Incorporated, 1999.)

After the flap is repositioned onto the dry stromal bed, it should be moistened on the surface and floated into position with a small amount of gentle irrigation under the flap. Forceful or prolonged irrigation can draw fluid and debris from the cul-de-sac into the interface by eddy currents. A "Fountain Cannula" (designed by Howard V. Gimbel) with a central port promotes flushing from the center to the periphery of the flap. A dripping wet Merocel sponge can then be used to gently express the fluid starting from the hinge then stroking away from the center. The physiological action will remove any remaining fluid. Touching or stroking the flap with anyting more than a delicate touch with a soaking wet sponge when it is floating can lead to stretching of the flap, resulting in wrinkles.

The Nidek laser has slit illumination, which is helpful for inspection of the flap for wrinkles at the end of surgery. The surgeon should be aware of the normal appearance of the flap following repositioning. The epithelial surface of the flap may have a peau-d'orange appearance due to surface irregularities of the sponge on which it rests during the ablation. These dimples, as well as epithelial wrinkles from slight folds in the flap when it is turned, will usually disappear shortlywithout additional manipulation. Wrinkles in the flap stroma may be identified using retroillumination intraoperatively, as well as postoperatively at the slit lamp using retroillumination and retinal reflected light (Figure 5-14). If wrinkles are seen intraoperatively, the flap can be refloated and smoothed using a wet sponge (Table 5-8). Wrinkles located at the flap edge may be ironed out with gentle traction using a dry Weck-cel sponge (Solan Ophthalmics, Jacksonville, Fla) dragged in a centripetal direction. Care must be taken to avoid excessive irrigation and manipulation of the flap, which can result in flap edema, stretching, epithelial keratitis, or epithelial disruption.

Table 5-8		
Wrinkled Flap Intraoperatively		
Possible Causes	• Improper flap positioning during the ablation • Excessive drying of the flap • Rough handling of the flap leading to stretching and microwrinkles when repositioning	
Results	• Wrinkles can lead to irregular astigmatism and visual disturbances	
Solutions	*Prevention* • Carefully lay the flap in a cupped position on a damp sponge during the ablation • Use a delicate touch with a wet sponge and begin smoothing at the hinge with subsequent motions away from the flap center • Do not leave any fluid under the flap *Management* • Smooth edge wrinkles by placing gentle traction with a dry Weck-cel sponge • Refloat into position with only a gentle manipulation • Epithelial wrinkles will often disappear without additional repositioning in a short time	

Interface Debris

Debris under the flap may result from poor fluid management (Table 5-9). If excessive irrigation is used, debris may be drawn up from the cul-de-sac. The slit beam of the Nidek laser allows for interface debris to be detected and removed prior to removing the speculum and drapes. If debris is appreciated at the slit lamp in the immediate postoperative assessment, the patient may be taken back to the operating suite for irrigation. If lipid, lint, or other debris is seen near the edge of the flap, a cannula can be passed under the flap only in the area of debris without lifting the entire flap. Centrally located debris necessitates that the entire flap be lifted and repositioned after the irrigation (Figure 5-15). Occasionally, a small stainless-steel particle may be seen in the flap interface. These particles may originate from the blade and may be quite difficult to remove, as they are usually imbedded in the undersurface of the flap. They do not typically cause any visual symptoms and do not need to be removed if they are off the visual axis.

Prolonged or repeated irrigation of the entire flap should be avoided, because it can lead to tissue swelling and retraction of the flap edges. Minimizing the time of irrigation will avoid stromal and flap hydration (which increase the risk of poor adherence).

Flap Edema

Flap edema is usually the result of prolonged manipulations and/or irrigation (Table 5-10). Flap edema can result in retraction, which may require that the flap be stretched into place using a dry sponge tip while stabilizing the eye with a

Table 5-9

Interface Debris

Possible Causes	• Poor fluid management drawing debris from cul-de-sac • Lint from sponge • Particles from microkeratome • Debris from the cannula, syringe, or bottle
Results	• Flap needs to be irrigated peripherally or possibly refloated if noted centrally
Solutions	*Prevention* • Irrigate and wipe cul-de-sac to remove mucous and debris prior to microkeratome pass • Avoid excess fluid on the surgical field • Carefully inspect microkeratome prior to each use • Carefully clean and rinse with clean water all reusable cannulas • Use disposable syringes *Management* • Inspect the interface and flap carefully prior to removing drapes and speculum • Edge irrigation may be used for peripheral debris • Lift flap and reposition after irrigation for centrally located debris

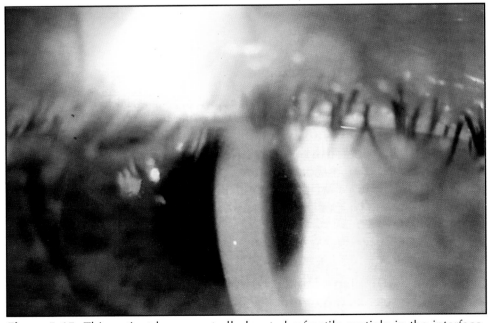

Figure 5-15. This patient has a centrally located refractile particle in the interface. (Reprinted with permission from Gimbel HV, Anderson Penno EE. *LASIK Complications: Prevention and Management.* Thorofare, NJ: SLACK Incorporated, 1999.)

Table 5-10	
Flap Edema	
Possible Causes	• Prolonged flap manipulation • Excessive irrigation
Result	• Flap edge retraction
Solutions	*Prevention* • Minimize handling of flap • Minimize irrigation under the flap *Management* • Attempt to gently stretch flap into place with a dry sponge as it begins to adhere • Sutures may be necessary in some cases

Thornton ring. When replacing edematous flaps and areas of loose epithelium are present, in rare cases sutures may be required to avoid a wide gutter around the flap and possible shifting of the flap in the early postoperative period.

Flap Shrinkage

In contrast to the flap retraction that can result from edema, flap shrinkage may be due to excessive drying before repositioning. To avoid prolonged delays, the patient should be in good position, and the laser should be armed prior to turning the flap (Table 5-11). We routinely measure the time between turning the flap and ablation; this interval is usually 10 to 15 seconds (Figure 5-16). As experience is gained, this interval is shortened (see Figures 4-1a and b).

Again, if significant shrinkage occurs and the flap cannot be stretched out because of reasons such as loose epithelium, then sutures should be placed to adequately position the flap and keep it in place (see Patient Example 8).

Flap Stretching

This complication is caused by excessive manipulation of the flap. It is essential to use a light touch with a soaking wet sponge when performing any smoothing maneuvers as the flap is repositioned. If the epithelium is loose or has been shifted by the microkeratome, the smoothing maneuver using wiping may stretch the epithelium into folds or stretch it over the edge of the flap. If this occurs, the epithelium should be gently repositioned. When the epithelium is very loose, the wet sponge should only touch rather than wipe. In rare cases, redundant epithelium may need to be trimmed away. After the epithelium is in place, a contact lens may be used as a bandage and left in place for a few hours or 1 to 2 days if necessary for a case with a large area of loose epithelium (Table 5-12).

Intraoperative Bleeding

While intraoperative hemorrhage does not pose a serious risk, it can be a nuisance. Patients with superficial corneal pannus related to long-term soft contact

Table 5-11

Flap Shrinkage

Possible Causes	• Excess drying due to delays in surgical technique
Results	• Necessitates stretching and/or sutures
Solutions	*Prevention* • Plan carefully so that the patient is centered at the laser and in good position prior to turning flap *Management* • Attempt to gently stretch flap into position • If necessary, sutures may be placed

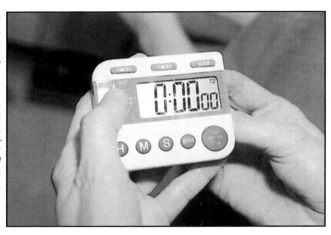

Figure 5-16. Routine measurement of the time between turning the flap and ablation. This interval is usually 10 to 15 seconds. As experience is gained, this interval is shortened. (Reprinted with permission from Gimbel HV, Anderson Penno EE. *LASIK Complications: Prevention and Management.* Thorofare, NJ: SLACK Incorporated, 1999.)

Table 5-12

Flap Stretching

Possible Causes	• Prolonged manipulation • Excessive force during smoothing or positioning maneuvers
Results	• Difficulty in positioning flap and/or epithelium • Visually significant striae
Solutions	*Prevention* • Minimize flap manipulations • Use a light touch with a soaking wet sponge when smoothing or positioning the flap *Management* • Gently reposition • Trim redundant epithelium • Place a contact lens as necessary

Table 5-13
Intraoperative Bleeding

Possible Causes	• Superficial corneal pannus • Larger flap size (Hansatome)
Results	• Delays in ablation due to the need to remove blood from the stromal bed • Additional steps may be needed to remove interface blood
Solutions	*Prevention* • A Chayet or Gimbel-Chayet sponge may be positioned to wick blood away from the hinge area *Management* • Pause the ablation and wick excess blood away from the bed if necessary • Irrigate the bed and gently wipe away any excess blood at edges after ablation • Irrigate any blood remaining in the interface and milk it from the flap edge using a damp sponge or the shaft of a cannula

(Reprinted with permission from Gimbel HV, Anderson Penno EE. LASIK Complications: Prevention and Management. Thorofare, NJ: SLACK Incorporated, 1999.)

lens use will be more prone to intraoperative bleeding (Table 5-13). The use of the Hansatome or other microkeratomes that make a large flap will more likely result in bleeding due to the larger flap size. To avoid blood on the stromal bed, a moistened Gimbel-Chayet sponge drain is used (Figures 5-17a through c). The sponge is placed so that any bleeding is wicked away from the flap edge. This sponge also serves to keep the flap from drying during the ablation and keeps it out of the debris and lipid-laden tears in the conjunctival cul-de-sac.

Should blood enter the stromal bed, the ablation should be paused. The blood should be carefully wicked away with a sponge, and the surface of the bed should be wiped with a spatula. Once the ablation is completed, any blood around the edges of the bed should be irrigated and/or gently wiped prior to laying the flap in place. A small film of remaining blood can be removed by irrigating under the flap and milking it from the edges using a sponge or the shaft of a cannula.

Epithelial Complications

Loose epithelium is most often encountered intraoperatively as the microkeratome makes its pass (Figure 5-18a and b, and Patient Example 19). Occasionally, a portion of epithelium will be dragged away from the underlying tissue. This most commonly occurs superiorly, and the loose epithelium should be carefully smoothed into place after the flap has been repositioned. Special care should be taken to avoid getting epithelial debris in the flap interface. First, a moist spear should be used to maneuver epithelium into place. Occasionally a dry Weck-cel

Figure 5-17a. The Chayet sponge. (Reprinted with permission from Gimbel HV, Anderson Penno EE. *LASIK Complications: Prevention and Management.* Thorofare, NJ: SLACK Incorporated, 1999.)

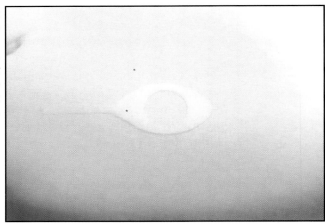

Figure 5-17b. The Chayet is cut as demonstrated. (Reprinted with permission from Gimbel HV, Anderson Penno EE. *LASIK Complications: Prevention and Management.* Thorofare, NJ: SLACK Incorporated, 1999.)

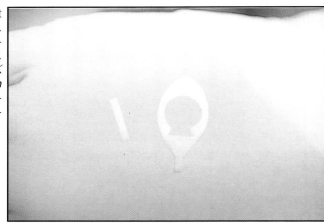

Figure 5-17c. The Gimbel-Chayet eye drain is used so that it can be placed (as demonstrated) with the edges of the sponge tucked under the edges of the hinge. In this way, any extraneous bleeding will be absorbed and will not flow onto the stromal bed and interfere with the ablation.

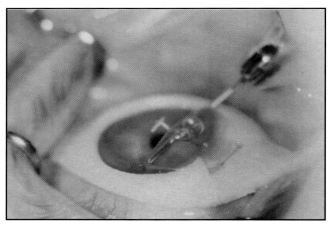

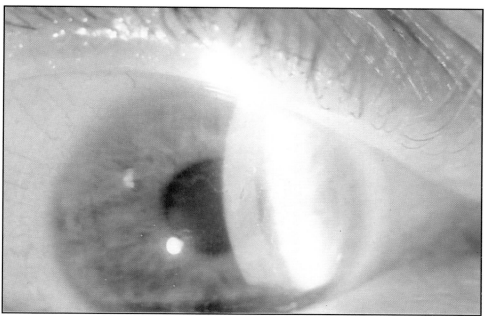

Figure 5-18a. This patient has a central area of loose and torn epithelium (see Patient Example 13). (Reprinted with permission from Gimbel HV, Anderson Penno EE. *LASIK Complications: Prevention and Management.* Thorofare, NJ: SLACK Incorporated, 1999.)

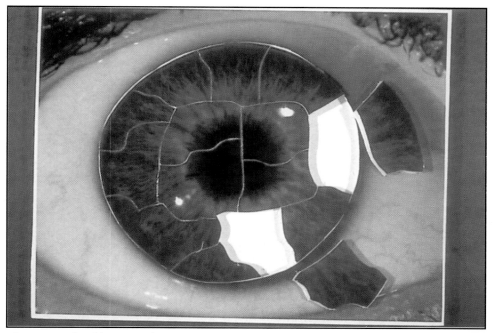

Figure 5-18b. If loose and torn epithelium is encountered, it should be replaced just like a jigsaw puzzle. (Reprinted with permission from Gimbel HV, Anderson Penno EE. *LASIK Complications: Prevention and Management.* Thorofare, NJ: SLACK Incorporated, 1999.)

sponge is needed to gently move stretched epithelium back into position. In some cases, one is unable to properly reposition the loose or torn epithelium and it must be removed. The gentian violet marks can be lost if the epithelium is disrupted in that location, which highlights the importance of marking at more than one site (as illustrated in Figure 5-8).

Use of preoperative anesthetic drops and other topical medications should be limited, as prolonged and over use may lead to softening and overhydration of the epithelium. Furthermore, the presence of basement membrane dystrophies or recurrent erosions should be noted preoperatively, as these patients are at risk for epithelial complications.

Some surgeons test epithelial adherence at the slit lamp during assessment with a dry Q-tip (Chesebrough-Pond USA Co., Greenwich, Conn) after instilling proparacaince hydrochloride. If significant epithelial looseness or basement membrane dystrophy is detected, PRK may be a better option (if appropriate). If more than 50% of the epithelium is disrupted on the first eye, there is a high likelihood of similar disruption on the second eye. Therefore, in these situations PRK is offered for the second eye. In these cases, the patient is often more satisfied with the PRK eye since epithelial irregularities with LASIK can delay visual recovery by days to weeks (see Patient Example 36).

Corneal abrasions have been reported as a result of improper draping, corneal marking, or placement/removal of the speculum. Particular care should be taken when placing or removing the speculum, especially in a patient who may be more nervous than the average. Careful instructions for the patient to keep both eyes open may help to avoid squeezing during this maneuver. Warning the patient that the lids are not anesthetized and that he or she may feel some pressure sensations on the lids will help to avoid sudden head or eye movements. Abrasions at the end of the procedure occur only rarely and can be managed with a bandage contact lens if necessary (Table 5-14). An improperly seated microkeratome blade or a blade that is not moving may also result in an abrasion. Care must also be taken when turning the flap because the forceps can damage the epithelium (Figure 5-19).

Patients are instructed to wear eye shields until they get home, and then while sleeping or napping for the first week. This helps to protect the epithelium and flap from inadvertent eye rubbing. A bandage contact lens may be placed in patients with significant epithelial disruption. The contact will provide pain relief and may avoid further loosening of the epithelium due to eyelid movement. If possible, patching should be avoided because the eye can dry and the flap can stick to the eyelid and then be easily dislodged. However, in rare cases, it may be needed if the patient is unable to tolerate a contact lens or the contact lens does not stay in place (see Patient Example 13).

Patching/Shielding/Bandage Contact Lenses

As a general rule, patching should be avoided. Patching may, in fact, lead to a dislodged flap if the epithelium is edematous or disturbed. Bandage contact lenses are indicated in cases of epithelial disruption.

Table 5-14
Epithelial Complications

Possible Causes
- Excessive preoperative drops
- Improper draping
- Rough corneal marking
- Patient squeezing eyes when placing/removing micro-keratome
- Failure of the blade to move
- Basement membrane dystrophy
- Forceps damage

Results
- Abrasions
- Loose epithelium
- Loss of gentian violet marks

Solutions

Prevention
- Limit preoperative drops
- Instruct patients not to squeeze eyes and to look straight ahead while inserting and removing drapes and speculum
- Use a gentle touch when marking or handling the flap
- Warn patients with basement membrane dystrophy that they are at higher risk for epithelial complications
- If appropriate, consider PRK for the second eye if significant loose epithelium was encountered on first eye

Management
- Carefully smooth the epithelium into position
- Occasionally the epithelium will stretch and excess tags need to be removed
- A contact lens may be placed in select cases with severe epithelial disruption
- Moisture chambers should be used in all patients

(Reprinted with permission from Gimbel HV, Anderson Penno EE. LASIK Complications: Prevention and Management. Thorofare, NJ: SLACK Incorporated, 1999.)

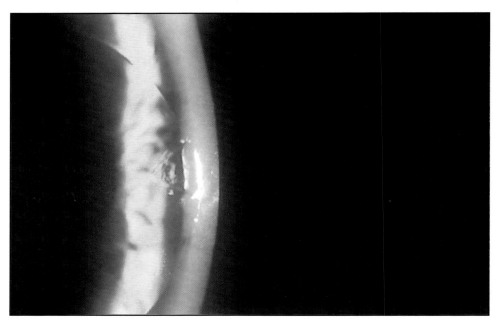

Figure 5-19. This photograph demonstrates the type of epithelial disruption that occurs when forceps are used in handling the flap. (Reprinted with permission from Gimbel HV, Anderson Penno EE. *LASIK Complications: Prevention and Management.* Thorofare, NJ: SLACK Incorporated, 1999.)

In localities with an arid climate, all patients should be discharged with clear plastic shields taped airtight to the skin, providing a high humidity environment to the eye in the early postoperative period when the anesthetic is reducing the normal blink reflex and reflex tearing is not normal (Figures 5-20a and b). These serve a dual purpose as moisture chambers and also as protection from inadvertent eye rubbing. Patients are instructed to leave them on until they return home, when napping or sleeping for the remainder of the first postoperative day, and at bedtime for 1 week. This routine should also be used for patients with exophthalmos, lagophthalmos, poor blinking, and any other high risk condition. We recommend use of a shield routinely.

Decentration

Decentered ablations can lead to irregular astigmatism and cause symptoms of glare, night vision problems, ghosting, and diplopia (Table 5-15 and Patient Example 25). The most important element leading to good centration is helping the patient remain alert and not lose focus on maintaining steady fixation. The patient must first be positioned comfortably and centered with regard to the target. Sedation should be minimized and avoided unless absolutely necessary, as this might make it more difficult for the patient to concentrate on maintaining fixation. As systems may vary, the surgeon should be familiar with the target of the particular laser in use so that instructions can be given appropriately. It is helpful to let the patient know that the target may become blurry after lifting the flap and

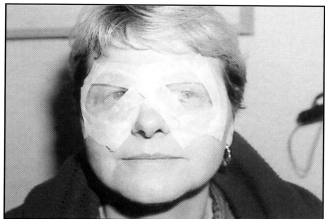

Figure 5-20a. This photograph shows the older style of moisture chambers used postoperatively. (Reprinted with permission from Gimbel HV, Anderson Penno EE. *LASIK Complications: Prevention and Management.* Thorofare, NJ: SLACK Incorporated, 1999.)

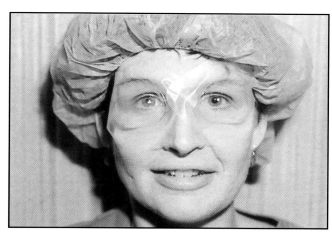

Figure 5-20b. The newer type has a self-adhesive cuff that aids in application. (Reprinted with permission from Gimbel HV, Anderson Penno EE. *LASIK Complications: Prevention and Management.* Thorofare, NJ: SLACK Incorporated, 1999.)

Table 5-15
Decentration

Possible Causes	• Poor patient fixation due to nervousness or oversedation • Difficulty seeing target due to blurred vision (especially in high corrections) • Improper use of Thornton ring
Results	• Loss of BCVA • Irregular astigmatism • Night vision problems • Ghosting, glare
Solutions	*Prevention* • Careful preoperative and intraoperative instructions as to fixation target, to keep both eyes open, not to squeeze fellow eye shut, and not to move arms and legs, as this causes the head to move • Warn about any sounds or smells that may startle patients • Careful use of Thornton ring in select patients *Management* • As described in Chapter 7

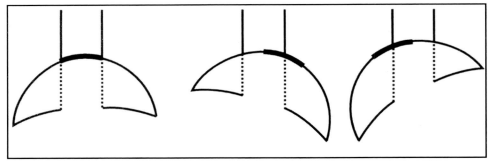

Figure 5-21. Thornton ring. Improper use of a Thornton ring can result in decentration. With eye rotation, the cornea moves more than the pupil or limbus. To avoid corneal rotation, centration should be checked by gently lifting and replacing the Thornton ring, as described in the text. (Reprinted with permission from Gimbel HV, Anderson Penno EE. *LASIK Complications: Prevention and Management.* Thorofare, NJ: SLACK Incorporated, 1999.)

to coach the patient to continue to look at the center of the target—this helps to alleviate anxiety. It may also be helpful to warn patients about the sounds and smells of the microkeratome and laser so that they aren't startled. Some surgeons like to tell the patient the length of the ablation and repeatedly announce the remaining time. These techniques are helpful with all patients but may be particularly important when dealing with a nervous patient. All of these techniques are aimed at keeping the patient relaxed and helping to optimize fixation.

If fixation is hard to maintain in spite of careful patient positioning and instruction, the ablation should be paused. It may be helpful to stabilize the patient's eye with a Thornton or Fine-Thornton ring while ablation is continued. It may also help to instruct the patient to keep the fellow eye open under the shield and not to squeeze the fellow eye shut. When placing the Thornton ring, begin by instructing the patient to fixate on the target. Hold the head steady and adjust the focus so that only slight downward pressure on the eye will bring the eye in perfect focus. The Thornton ring should be placed with only a slight downward pressure; rotation of the globe while placing the ring must be avoided, because this may result in a decentration (Figure 5-21). Centration can be checked by gently lifting the Thornton ring, checking to see if the eye moves, and then replacing it once centration is ensured.

A decentration may cause enough visual aberration that a retreatment will be necessary. Retreatment strategies for symptomatic decentration will be discussed in Chapter 7.

REFERENCE

1. Slade SG. LASIK complications and their management. Free cap, thin and perforated corneal flaps. In: Machat JJ, ed. *Excimer Laser Refractive Surgery: Practice and Principles.* Thorofare, NJ: SLACK Incorporated; 1996.

6

Early Postoperative Complications: 24 to 48 Hours

There are major and minor complications that may be observed in the early postoperative period following LASIK. It is customary to schedule a postoperative exam during this period to screen for these early complications.

PAIN

One of the advantages of LASIK is that the recovery is rapid and pain is usually not a major issue. Patients are counseled to expect watering, sensitivity to light, some gritty or foreign body sensation, and possibly a small amount of discomfort that should resolve rather quickly. If needed, patients may take non-narcotic analgesics, such as acetaminophen. Narcotics should not be necessary, and any patient who complains of significant pain needs assessment at the slit lamp. Pain is usually indicative of flap or epithelial disruption, and management will vary depending on the underlying cause.

It is not uncommon for patients undergoing enhancement procedures that lift the flap rather than recutting a flap to remark that there is more discomfort than was noted on the primary treatment. This is most likely due to irregularities in the epithelium where the flap was dissected and from epithelium that was swept back from the flap edge before the flap was replaced to avoid epithelial ingrowth. Small

Table 6-1	
Early Postoperative Pain (24 to 48 hours)	
Possible Causes	• Uncomplicated LASIK may result in epiphora, photophobia, foreign body sensation • Epithelial disruption (loose epithelium or abrasion) • Shifted flap
Results	• Patient anxiety • Need for analgesia
Solutions	*Prevention* • Preoperative counseling with regard to patient expectations; warn patients that they may experience foreign body sensation that may be worse with enhancements *Management* • Severe or persistent pain (>24 hours) should result in a slit lamp exam • Contact lens can be placed if needed • Recommend non-narcotic analgesia • Liberal use of artificial tears • Reassurance

areas of loose epithelium may be present from these maneuvers. A contact lens is generally not necessary and the patients should be reassured that it is not uncommon to have slightly more discomfort after enhancements. Severe pain or pain that occurs after the immediate postoperative period may indicate a shifted flap, and these patients should be examined at the slit lamp (Table 6-1).

EPITHELIAL COMPLICATIONS

The most common intraoperative and postoperative complication associated with LASIK is loose epithelium intraoperatively.[1] Management of these cases is the same as for loose epithelium encountered intraoperatively (see Table 5-14). A bandage contact lens can be placed after smoothing loose epithelium into place to avoid further disruption and as a pain control measure. Epithelial tags should be removed at the slit lamp prior to placing a contact. In the postoperative follow-up period, the contact lens should be left in place until the epithelium has completely healed. Premature removal of the contact lens may lead to peeling of the epithelium during removal of the lens.[1] The contact lens serves both as a protection to the epithelium and for pain control. Patients are advised not to rub their eyes and to continue using antibiotic/corticosteroid drops and copious viscous lubricants. Pressure patching is generally contraindicated due to the risk of shifting of the flap.

INFECTIONS

Infections following LASIK are extremely rare.[2-9] However, because bacterial keratitis can be sight-threatening, every measure should be taken to prevent this

Table 6-2
Postoperative Keratitis

Possible Causes	• Infections (rare) • Toxic (Sands of the Sahara)
Results	• Pain • Blurred vision
Solutions	*Prevention* • Careful cleaning of all cannulas and syringes using fresh sterile distilled water for ultrasound cleaning, washing, and rinsing • Careful clearing and inspections of microkeratome assembly and blade • Treatment of blepharitis preoperatively • Sterile technique • Avoid excess irrigation intraoperatively • Prophylactic postoperative topical antibiotic/steroid solution • Recommend no swimming or hot tubs for 2 weeks postoperatively *Management* • Patent steroid drops every 1 to 2 hours in noninfectious cases • Topical NSAID drops • Topical antibiotics • Close observation • Lifting the flap and scraping the bed and undersurface of the cap in severe cases

complication. Despite the low risk, sterile intraoperative techniques in addition to the postoperative use of antibiotics is recommended. Patients with blepharitis should be adequately treated prior to LASIK. Preventive measures include avoiding excessive irrigation intraoperatively to prevent debris from the cul-de-sac from entering into the interface (Table 6-2).

The organisms isolated from the rare cases reported in the literature include Streptococcus,[3] Staphylococcus,[4] and Nocardia.[5] Some infections were also culture negative.[6-7] Clinical presentation range from corneal infiltrates to lamellar abscess formation in the interface.[4,8] Topical intensive antibiotic therapy is the preferred treatment. In severe cases and in cases of abscess formation, lifting the flap, scraping, culture and sensitivities, and irrigation of the stromal bed with antibiotics has been advocated.[2,4] Reactivation of herpes simplex virus (HSV) keratitis has also been reported following LASIK, therefore history of HSV should be considered a contraindication to surgery.[9]

DIFFUSE LAMELLAR KERATITIS

Diffuse lamellar keratitis (DLK), first described as the Sands of Sahara syndrome, is a noninfectious inflammation involving the interface.[10] DLK typically

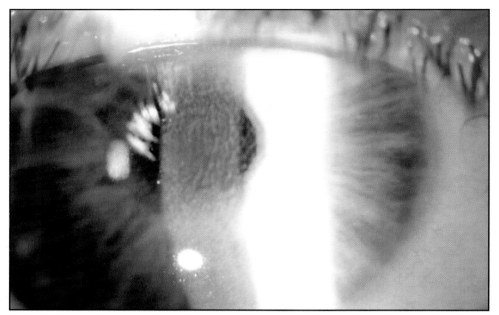

Figure 6-1. Typical granular appearance of interface inflammation in DLK.

presents 1 to 5 days after LASIK. Patients may have decreased visual acuity, for-eign body sensation, or photophobia.[10] Slit lamp examination reveals fine granu-larity limited to the interface (Figure 6-1).[10] Inflammation is typically diffuse and confined to the interface with no flap or stromal extension.[10,11] The anterior chamber is usually quiet.[10] More severe forms may present with the typical shift-ing sand dune-like pattern, and severe untreated inflammation may cause the flap to melt.

Four grades of DLK have been proposed.[12] Grade 1 includes the presence of white granular cells in the periphery of the interface. Grade 2 is defined by the presence of the same cells in the center and/or the periphery of the interface involving the visual axis. Grade 3 involves dense aggregates of white clumped cells centrally with relative clearing peripherally. Grade 4 involves scarring and stromal melting.

The etiology of DLK is unknown. Various etiologies have been proposed and it is possible that DLK may result from a number of possible causes (see Table 6-2). Contamination from the microkeratome, gloves, debris from the eyelid including meibomian gland secretions, and eyelid-related or irrigation fluid-related bacterial endotoxin have all been implicated as etiological factors.[8,9,11,13] There is an increased incidence in patients with large patches of loose epithelium intraoperatively.[2]

Patients with Grades 1 and 2 DLK are treated with intensive topical steroids with topical antibiotic coverage.[10,14] Most of these cases tend to resolve within 2 to 4 weeks. In Grades 3 and 4, the flap should be lifted and the granular material should be scraped off the flap and the stromal bed as soon as possible.[12,14] Some surgeons advocate irrigating the interface with steroids as a preventive measure against DLK (see Patient Examples 19 to 22).[15]

Preliminary data from a rabbit model in which a LASIK flap is created indicate that endotoxin causes lamellar inflammation with dose response effect (Gimbel et al, unpublished data) (Figures 6-2a and b). Further studies demonstrate that polymixin, which binds endotoxin, has some effect of reducing lamellar inflammation when placed directly on the stromal bed intraoperatively. Inflammase did not appear to reduce inflammation when placed intraoperatively, but when a steroid is used postoperatively, it has the overall effect of reducing inflammation regardless of the endotoxin dose. The preliminary data from this unpublished study of lamellar keratitis in a rabbit model indicate that while there is no strong evidence for the routine use of intraoperative steroid or polymixin, routine postoperative treatment should include a topical steroid.

INTERFACE DEBRIS

Introduction of foreign materials into the interface may occur during LASIK. Talc, fibers from the Merocel spongel, mucus, or oil from the tear film or the cul-de-sac, lashes, and metal shavings from the microkeratome blade have been reported (Figures 6-3a and b).[2,16] Some foreign material in the interface, such as metal filings or tiny lipid or mucous particles, usually do not cause inflammation or surface irregularities and are best left untreated. Peripheral inert substances should also be left untreated. However, irregularity of the flap interface due to inflammation from foreign material such as talc or fibers can lead to loss of the BCVA secondary to irregular astigmatism. Epithelial debris in the interface or epithelial ingrowth from the edge may also cause stromal melt.[17,18] Therefore, patients who present with inflammation from interface debris or epithelial ingrowth should also have them removed and irrigated. Foreign bodies in the pupillary zone or multiple central debris should also be removed.[19]

Debris at the edge of the flap can be removed by placing a cannula under the flap edge in the location of the debris. If the debris is located centrally, the flap will need to be lifted entirely, scraped, irrigated, and repositioned. Excessive irrigation may carry debris onto the stromal bed from the cul-de-sac. Minimizing irrigation and careful inspection intraoperatively will help reduce the need to take patients back to surgery for this complication (see Table 5-9).

WRINKLES AND FOLDS

Wrinkles in the stromal tissue of the flap are easily identified on the first postoperative day by retroillumination (Table 6-3, Figures 6-4a and b). Predisposing factors include prolonged surgery time, exophthalmos, lagophthalmos, excessive interface irrigation, stromal hydration and poor flap adherence, and lateral canthotomy with temporary poor blinking, as the local anesthetic may affect the orbicularis.[20] Wrinkles also seem to be more common in highly myopic patients. Adherence should be tested with the striae test. Some surgeons wait up to 4 minutes after the flap is in position to remove the speculum. If the surgery proceeds

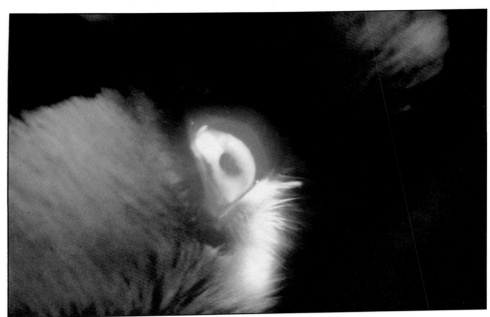

Figure 6-2a. Mild lamellar keratitis in a rabbit model.

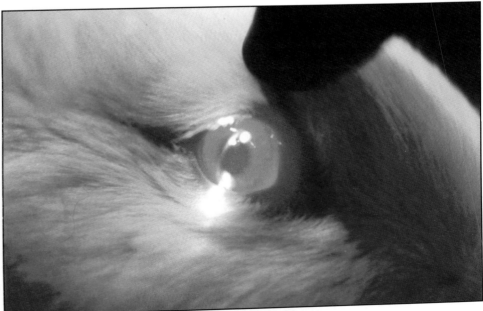

Figure 6-2b. Severe lamellar keratitis in a rabbit model.

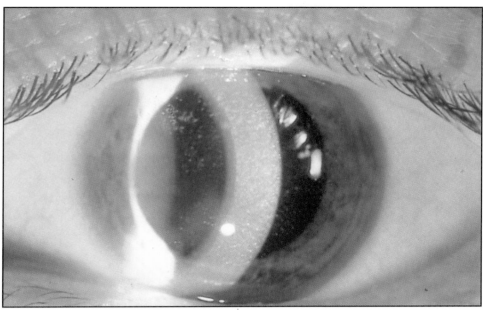

Figure 6-3a. Interface debris. This patient underwent bilateral LASIK elsewhere and was noted to have lipid-like particles in the interface postoperatively. (Reprinted with permission from Gimbel HV, Anderson Penno EE. *LASIK Complications: Prevention and Management.* Thorofare, NJ: SLACK Incorporated, 1999.)

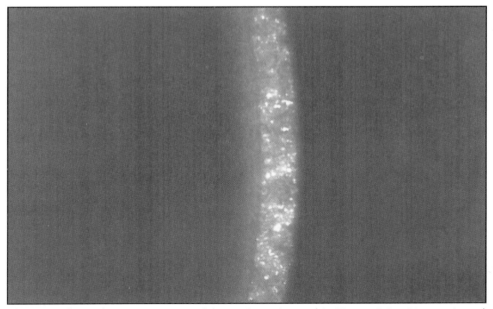

Figure 6-3b. Higher power view of the patient pictured in Figure 6-3a. He continued to have good vision (20/15[-3] OD and 20/15[-1] OS uncorrected) throughout the post-operative period. The patient was maintained on a tapering antibiotic/steriod combination and was continuing to improve at the time of last consultation. (Reprinted with permission from Gimbel HV, Anderson Penno EE. *LASIK Complications: Prevention and Management.* Thorofare, NJ: SLACK Incorporated, 1999.)

Table 6-3

Wrinkled and Shifted Flap Postoperatively

Possible Causes	• Squeezing lids • Eye rubbing • Poor blink • Lid or orbital abnormalities resulting in poor wetting • Lateral canthotomy • Loose epithelium leading to poor flap adherence • Poor adherence • Postoperative trauma
Results	• Necessity for repositioning • Risk of epithelial edema, abrasions, epithelial ingrowth • Possibly will need sutures
Solutions	*Prevention* • Careful attention to any lid or orbit abnormalities preoperatively • Check adherence with the striae test at the end of the case • Moisture chambers in all patients • Counsel patient to avoid squeezing lids and to wear moisture chambers for 24 hours and then every night for 1 week postoperatively *Management* • Tips of dry sponges may be used to stretch flap after it adheres to stromal bed (if the epithelium is intact) • Suture flap edges in cases with persistent wrinkles and/or loose epithelium • Clear off epithelium from flap edges if shifted flap ≥ 24 hours postoperatively • Verify correct position by examining the gutter width circumferentially

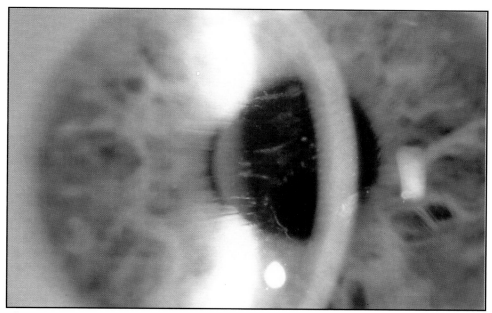

Figure 6-4a. This photograph demonstrates preoperative buttonhole and shifted flaps that were encountered (see Patient Example 6). (Reprinted with permission from Gimbel HV, Anderson Penno EE. *LASIK Complications: Prevention and Management.* Thorofare, NJ: SLACK Incorporated, 1999.)

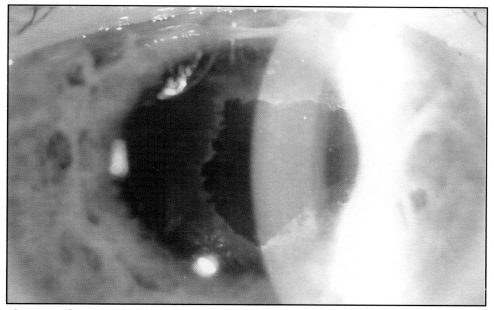

Figure 6-4b. This photograph demonstrates postoperative buttonhole and shifted flaps that were encountered (see Patient Example 6). (Reprinted with permission from Gimbel HV, Anderson Penno EE. *LASIK Complications: Prevention and Management.* Thorofare, NJ: SLACK Incorporated, 1999.)

quickly and stromal hydration is minimized, good flap adherence should occur in 1 to 2 minutes. However, in spite of good adherence, the flap can shift and cause a wrinkle if the surface dries and the eyelid friction is too great.

Peripheral wrinkles not in the visual axis and not affecting the BCVA may be left alone. However, if the flap has wrinkles in the visual axis and the BCVA is reduced, then it should be repositioned. In cases where the patient presents on the first or second postoperative day, a Sinsky hook is used to break the epithelial bonds at the flap edge and a spatula is used to reflect the flap. If the wrinkles are localized to one quadrant of the flap, then only that area needs to be refloated. If the wrinkles are central, then the entire flap needs to be refloated and repositioned. Any epithelium that may have migrated onto the exposed stromal bed is wiped back or scraped with a Paton spatula. Careful management of the epithelium is important to avoid epithelial ingrowth.

There are two techniques that may aid in removing flap wrinkles.[20] After the initial smoothing of the flap into position, but prior to the time the flap begins to adhere firmly to the bed, the tip of a dry Merocel sponge may be used to stretch the flap and help appose the gutter. The epithelium must be strongly adhered to the flap or the loose epithelium must be removed for this maneuver to work. The wrinkles will still be visible in the epithelium at the end of repositioning but will resolve by the next day. Careful inspection with the laser slit beam or at the slit lamp may help to discern the difference between stromal and epithelial wrinkles. An alternative technique, which is only rarely necessary, is to suture the flap edges to stretch the flap and remove wrinkles. The suture should ideally be a running 10-0 nylon antitorque suture, but interrupted sutures may be used as long as they are placed evenly throughout the entire circumference of the flap (Figure 6-5).

SHIFTED AND DISLODGED FLAPS

Shifted flaps occurred within the first 24 hours in 1.2% of our first 1000 cases reported,[22] and in 0.85% of cases reported by Stulting, et al.[23] Flap displacement may be caused by drying due to inadequate blinking, stromal edema from excessive irrigation, epithelial trauma, unstable free cap, or by rubbing (see Table 6-3).[21] Moisture chambers are mandatory after LASIK surgery (at least until the anesthetic wears off in low humidity climates). We have virtually eliminated shifted flaps by requiring the patients to wear moisture chambers following surgery.

Shifted flaps can be managed by carefully lifting the dislodged portion, cleaning epithelium from the stromal bed and edges of the bed, and refloating using the smoothing techniques described above for wrinkled flaps. Antitorque sutures are rarely needed to secure the flap. Prompt recognition and early surgical intervention in these cases typically results in a successful surgical outcome.[24]

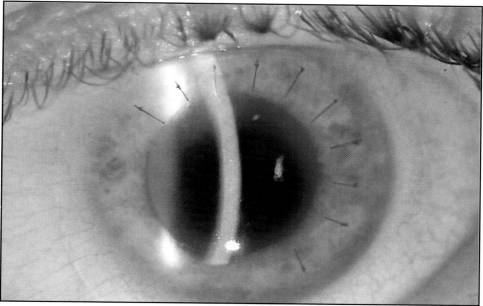

Figure 6-5. Flap sutures. This photgraph demonstrates a patient in whom sutures were used to stretch the flap and remove wrinkles (see Patient Example 21). (Reprinted with permission from Gimbel HV, Anderson Penno EE. *LASIK Complications: Prevention and Management.* Thorofare, NJ: SLACK Incorporated, 1999.)

DIFFUSE LAMELLAR KERATITIS

Damien C. Macaluso, MD, and Scott M. MacRae, MD

Introduction

As LASIK has become increasing popular among refractive surgeons, so has the recognition of the perplexing and potentially sight-threatening disorder of DLK. The early definitive diagnosis and treatment of this disorder are the key to avoiding irregular astigmatism, hyperopia, and devastating loss of BCVA that can result if this disorder is not promptly diagnosed and aggressively treated. In this chapter, we will outline some of the confusing terminology (Table 1) and potential causes, as well as review an aggressive treatment protocol that we have found to be very helpful in avoiding the sight-threatening complications associated with this disorder.

History

In November 1996, Maddox reported the initial cases of this entity when four patients who had LASIK on the same day developed DLK.[1] Additional cases were later reported by others in nonpeer-reviewed journals, and as presentations and

Table 1
Additional Terms Describing DLK

- Sands of Sahara (SOS) syndrome
- Shifting sands
- Sterile interface keratitis
- Lamellar keratitis
- Diffuse interlamellar keratitis (DIK)
- Nonspecific diffuse interlamellar keratitis (NSDIK)
- Interface Keratitis Interface inflammation after LASIK

courses at various ophthalmology meetings. The first peer-reviewed publication of this entity appeared in March 1998 by Smith and Maloney, who characterized 13 eyes with the disorder and called it DLK.[2] Additional reports have followed in an attempt to delineate potential etiologies, grade various stages of the condition, and outline treatment regimens.

Etiology: Multifactorial Causes

Since the initial reports of DLK, much speculation has revolved around the potential causes (Table 2). Initial reports consisted of cases occurring in clusters, and subsequent theories focused on contaminants introduced under the flap during surgery. This included any substance that came into contact with the interface, or residue on an instrument contacting the interface. Current theories as to the etiology are numerous.[3,4,5,6]

Anecdotal cases have been described in which many of these individual factors were not utilized during the procedure and could not possibly have contributed to the development of DLK. This suggested that no single agent is responsible for all cases of this syndrome and that the underlying etiology is likely multifactorial.

The antigenic endotoxin on gram-negative bacterial cell wall surfaces is capable of inciting an intense neutrophilic reaction. This lipopolysaccharide (LPS) unit is stable for the short cycles of steam sterilization used with most LASIK instruments. Holland, and subsequently Schumer, suggested that the sterilizer reservoirs might serve as a source for bacterial particles to accumulate (American Academy of Ophthalmology, Refractive Surgery Special Interest Group, Orlando, Fla October 1999). They hypothesized that the reservoirs may serve as a site where bacteria proliferate. The bacteria are killed by the sterilizer during sterilization, but the cellular particles such as the LPS (gram-negative bacteria) and peptidoglycan (gram-positive bacteria) may accumulate on the surgical instruments during the sterilization process. When the surgical instruments are used, the cellular particles get into the interface and stimulate a strong immunologic response. This mechanism may be responsible for multiple cases of DLK that occur from the same center in one day.

Table 2

Etiologies of Diffuse Lamellar Keratitis

Endogenous

- Meibomian gland secretions
- Bacterial components from eyelid margin*
- Transected corneal epithelial cells

- Overlying epithelial defects*
- Additional tear film debris
- Red blood cells

Exogenous

- Contaminants from instruments or sterilizers*
- Bacterial endotoxin*
- Nonsteroidal anti-inflammatory drops
- Lubricant or rust from microkeratome*
- Particulate matter from the drapes, gown, or gloves

- Balanced salt solution (BSS)
- Benzalkonium chloride
- Bacterial exotoxin*
- Povidone-iodine
- Excimer laser energy

* Indicates etiologies that the authors believe are more likely

Host Factors

We have noted a greater preponderance of interface keratitis in patients with atopic disease, including atopic dermatitis (eczema), chronic sinusitis, allergic rhinitis and reactive airway disease. This suggests that the host's immune system may play a role in the development of DLK.

The host's immune system may also react strongly to respond to anatomical abnormalities, such as an epithelial defect, to cause interface inflammation. In addition, we have also noted DLK in a patient who had a tight soft contact lens syndrome following LASIK.

While the etiology may be difficult to identify, the underlying pathophysiology is ultimately due to recruitment of polymorphonuclear leukocytes to the stromal interface. Presumably, these cells migrate in an immune response to an antigenic stimulus collecting in the interface. The nature, quantity, and duration of exposure to the antigen may influence this reaction. In addition, the host immune response and modulation of this response are likely significant factors.

Diagnosis

Differential

Careful slit lamp inspection reveals a characteristic appearance of DLK; however, other disorders may mimic this appearance. Familiarity with these other conditions may help aid in the correct diagnosis. Early recognition of a microbial keratitis in the postoperative period is essential. An infectious infiltrate may or may not result in decreased vision, but there is usually associated pain and photophobia. These same symptoms may occur with more severe grades of DLK. With microbial keratitis, the conjunctiva is usually inflamed with an accompanying ciliary flush and is often associated with a purulent discharge, especially in the later stages of infection. The white infiltrate associated with bacterial keratitis is mostly focal and may extend either anteriorly into the flap or posteriorly into the stromal bed.

In DLK, the infiltrate has a fine, rippled, powdery appearance confined to the interface, which does not extend anteriorly or posteriorly. The infiltrate may be sectoral or diffuse, but it does not appear as a single focus. If the diagnosis is in question, then lifting the flap and obtaining a specimen for culture and gram stain is prudent. At the same time, the interface can be thoroughly irrigated with BSS. Intense hourly topical antibiotics should then be initiated. If the gram stain reveals neutrophils and no bacteria, then one may consider focusing treatment more intensively for DLK while maintaining antibiotic coverage. Although a gram stain negative for bacteria may aid in the diagnosis, it does not totally exclude an early microbial keratitis. The patient's clinical course and cultures should be closely followed.

Aside from microbial keratitis, particulate matter deposited in the interface may appear similar to DLK. Endogenous substances such as meibomian gland secretions, red blood cells, or epithelium may be noted in the interface in the early postoperative period. Exogenous substances may also be deposited in the interface, such as debris from sponges, talc, lubricant or rust from the microkeratome, instrument debris, or other particulate matter. While many of these substances are theorized to incite DLK, we have observed that some of these substances may be present in the interface without any associated inflammation. For instance, we have reported on several cases of red blood cells in the interface,[6] which have been self-limited. When bleeding occurs in the flap at the time of surgery, it is helpful to note the location of the hemorrhage in the operative report. The day after surgery, we often observe a sectoral collection of cells in the interface where the hemorrhage occurred. These cells rapidly resorb over the next few days.

Symptoms

The symptoms of DLK are very similar to the symptoms experienced with other forms of keratitis. One important characteristic of DLK is that during the mild or early stages, the patient is often completely asymptomatic and the vision may be very good. With moderate or severe forms of DLK, patients exhibit varying degrees of redness, pain or irritation, photophobia, and decreased vision.

Signs

DLK often follows an uncomplicated LASIK as a barely perceptible peripheral interface haze on the first postoperative day (Figure 1). By the third to fourth postoperative day, the haze evolves into a faint white or tan colored powdery substance with a mixed granular and rippled appearance and progresses throughout the lamellar interface (Figure 2). The cells may be seen following a pattern that resembles the laser ablation profile or the chatter marks of the microkeratome. At this point, patients may experience a subjective decrease in vision, and occasionally describe symptoms of ocular irritation and photophobia. In most of these cases the

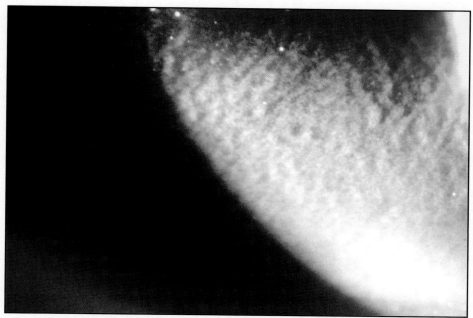

Figure 1. Fine white cells, accumulating in the interface, are distributed in a wave-like fashion at the periphery of the flap in stage 1.

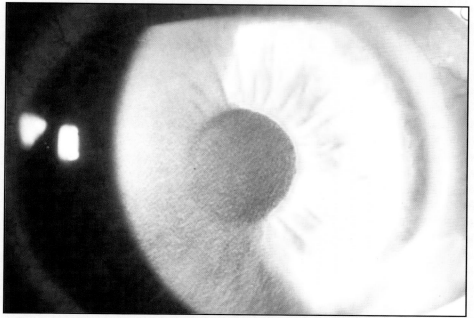

Figure 2. Granular or wave-like appearance of interface cells in the visual axis indicates stage 2. Note that the cells are over the pupillary area.

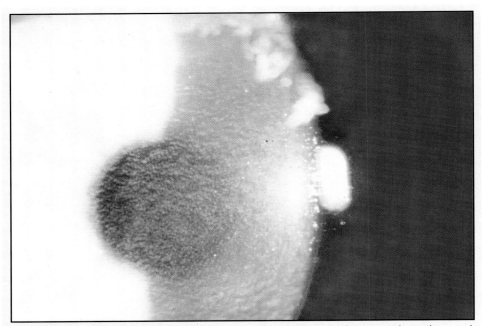

Figure 3. Increased density of interface cells in the visual axis with a clumped appearance is accompanied by a decrease in BCVA in stage 3.

haze gradually resolves and the rippled appearance fades within 1 to 2 weeks. In severe cases, the DLK worsens after the first postoperative day and the cells tend to aggregate centrally (Figure 3). Stromal melting may subsequently occur with fluid collecting in the lamellar interface and resultant stromal loss, and eventually permanent scarring (Figures 4a and b). At this point, patients may have associated conjunctival injection and a mild anterior chamber reaction. In the most severe cases, eyelid and periorbital edema and erythema may be present.

Grading/Staging

In an attempt to objectively quantify the degree of DLK, various individuals have proposed several staging or grading systems. Most of these classification systems are similar. However, since disparities do exist, we found it very helpful to give a detailed, narrative description of the signs and document any reduction in vision following a manifest refraction when describing a particular case. In more severe cases, we also found that computerized corneal topography can also be performed to document subtle changes in the corneal curvature caused by the inflammation.

Machat has characterized DLK by grades 1, 2, and 3.[7] Grade 1 represents the mildest stage in which the vision and refraction are unaffected and the patient is asymptomatic. The interface haze appears as a trace or mild PRK haze without associated loss of BCVA. Grade 2 is a moderate stage with BCVA reduced one to two lines, and the appearance of a centrally located moderate PRK haze. Grade 3 is more severe, and BCVA is reduced several lines (induced hyperopia and irregu-

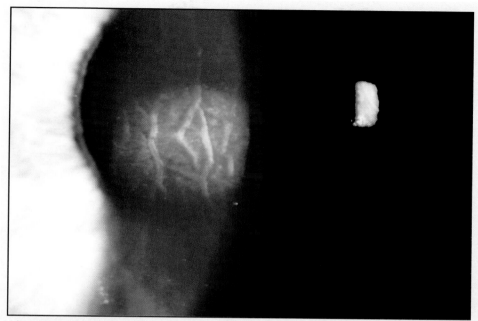

Figure 4a. Central focal scarring and large striae are present in the visual axis 4 months after LASIK in late stage 4, seen in slit lamp. This patient was not treated promptly with flap lifting and irrigation, or intensive topical or oral steroids.

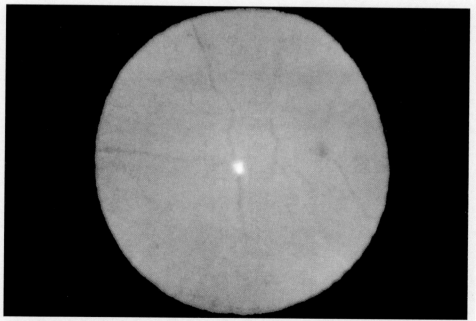

Figure 4b. Central focal scarring and large striae are present in the visual axis 4 months after LASIK in late stage 4, seen in retroillumination. This patient was not treated promptly with flap lifting and irrigation, or intensive topical or oral steroids.

lar astigmatism may also result). A dense central infiltrate is present, appearing similar to grade 4 PRK haze.

Hatsis has developed a similar classification system grading the disorder on four levels.[1] Grades I and II usually appear on day 1, but may be seen as late as day 3. It appears as a fine, diffuse interface infiltrate and the patient is asymptomatic with a visual acuity in the expected range of refraction. Grades III and IV are more severe forms in which the infiltrate is dense and tends to outline the ablation pattern and the chatter marks from the microkeratome. Loss of vision along with symptoms of ocular discomfort and photophobia may accompany the more severe stages.

Linebarger, Hardten, and Lindstrom have divided DLK into four stages[8] (Table 3). In stage 1, white, granular cells are present in the periphery of the lamellar flap with sparing of the visual axis. This stage is usually present on day 1 and may be seen as frequently as one in 25 to 50 cases.[8] In stage 2, the cells may migrate to the center of the flap and may still be present at the periphery. This stage may be seen on day 1, but more commonly this is seen as a progression of stage 1 and occurs on day 2 or 3. Stage 3 represents an aggregation of the white, clumped cells in the center of the flap with clearing in the periphery. Patients often describe a subjective haze and BCVA may be decreased one to two lines. The frequency of stage 3 may approach one in 500 cases.[8] Stage 4 is the most severe form, with permanent stromal scarring following fluid collection in the central lamella. Bullae formation may also result from variable degrees of stromal melt. This stage results in a more significant loss of BCVA associated with the development of irregular astigmatism and hyperopia. The incidence of this severity is approximately one in 5000 cases.[8]

These grading systems aid in defining the natural progression of this disorder. However, marked variability may exist in the time of onset, severity at presentation, location, and progression of DLK. The very mild stages are often present on day one, but may not be seen until a few days later. Many of these mild cases often resolve spontaneously over a period of a week without any sequelae. No factors have been identified that can accurately predict progression of DLK to the more severe stages so close follow-up is essential. Some of the more severe cases (stage/grade 3 and 4) may be seen as early as day 1, often making the differential diagnosis of DLK versus micobial keratitis more challenging. As many refractive surgeons may be unfamiliar with these various grading systems, we find it helpful to carefully document our clinical findings and correlate them with any loss of BCVA. The clinical findings then dictate the treatment regimen.

Laboratory Findings

Confirmation of the diagnosis of DLK is most often based on the history and the clinical presentation. If the diagnosis is uncertain and a microbial keratitis is considered in the differential, then obtaining a gram stain and culture of the infiltrate is appropriate. The presence of leukocytes without the presence of bacteria can be seen immediately on gram stain, and intervention may then be directed

Table 3

Treatment of Diffuse Lamellar Keratitis (Linebarger Staging)

Stage 1 (see Figure 1)

Clinical Findings	Treatment
• Fine, white cells distributed in a wave-like fashion at the periphery of the flap • No decrease in BCVA	• Prednisolone acetate or phosphate 1% every hour while awake • Follow-up 24 to 48 hours

Stage 2 (see Figure 2)

Clinical Findings	Treatment
• Granular or wave-like appearance of cells in the visual axis and possibly at the periphery • No decrease in BCVA • Patient may have ocular irritation or photophobia	• Prednisolone acetate 1% every hour while awake • Consider starting oral prednisone (60 to 80 mg po qid) if this appears on postoperative day 1 or patient has atopic or allergic disease • Follow-up 24 hours

Stage 3 (see Figure 3)

Clinical Findings	Treatment
• Increased density of cells in the visual axis, appears more clumped than wave-like • Patient may describe a subject haze • BCVA is decreased more than one line	• Prednisolone acetate 1% every hour while awake • Start oral prednisone (60 to 80 mg po qid) • Manually lift the flap and thoroughly irrigate

Stage 4 (see Figure 4)

Clinical Findings	Treatment
• Scarring and folds in the visual axis • BCVA is decreased • Irregular astigmatism, hyperopia	• Permanent scarring has resulted and no definitive late stage treatment is proven effective. Some improvement may occur over the next 6 to 12 months • Consider treating as stage 3 if progressive

toward treatment of DLK. Coverage with a broad-spectrum antibiotic is appropriate while awaiting culture results and the regimen may be adjusted depending on the patient's course.

Confocal Microscopy

In vivo data is also available for a DLK model in rabbits.[4] Confocal microscopy of the lamellar interface created by LASIK in rabbits has demonstrated focal pockets of debris with associated clusters of inflammatory cells. These cells are thought to be polymorphonuclear leukocytes.

Treatment

In mild cases, topical corticosteroids are the treatment of choice (see Table 3). We recommend the use of full strength topical steroids, such as prednisolone acetate or phosphate 1%, used every hour while awake for the first 24 to 48 hours for treatment of Linebarger stages 1 and 2 (no decreased vision or clumping of cells centrally). The continuation of a broad-spectrum topical flouroquinolone antibiotic is appropriate. Patients are seen the following day to ensure that the inflammation has not worsened. If the condition has improved, then the topical steroids are tapered slowly over the following week. Most of the cases will start to improve by postoperative day 2 to 4 without affecting vision.

In more severe cases, cells may aggregate centrally under the flap and BCVA is reduced (Linebarger stage 3). If the inflammation has progressed to the point where the patient has lost two or more lines of best-corrected vision, a more aggressive approach is indicated. We advocate manually lifting the flap and thoroughly irrigating the stromal bed and undersurface of the flap with BSS. The flap lifting and irrigating limit the inflammatory reaction by removing and diluting the concentration of the inciting agent, as well as diluting chemical mediators of the inflammatory cascade that may lead to stromal melt and potential scarring. Continuation of intense hourly topical steroids and institution of oral corticosteroids is critical at this stage.

Oral Corticosteroids

We also strongly advocate the use of high-dose oral corticosteroids (prednisone 30 mg po bid in females and 40 mg po bid in males) in combination with intensive topical steroids to limit the immune system's response.[9] This strategy of a utilizing a short coarse of oral and topical corticosteroids has been used for years by dermatologists to treat severe atopic disease and other forms of hypersensitivity reactions, such as poison oak, and is very well tolerated. We have successfully treated 10 patients with this combination of high dose oral and intensive topical corticosteroids without any complications. Precaution should be taken when using oral steroids in diabetic patients or anyone with a contraindication to the use of oral corticosteroids.

Patients who respond at this stage tend to heal without any visible sequelae or limitation of BCVA. The object is to limit the inflammatory process early, in the first one to three days, and to prevent the development of stromal melting and irreversible scarring. Once this later stage has been reached less benefit is gained by lifting the flap and irrigating and a less than ideal visual outcome is likely. Vigorous debridement during this stage may result in extensive stromal volume

Table 4
Prevention of Diffuse Lamellar Keratitis

Instrumentation

- Clean and scrub instruments with mild detergent and rinse and soak in distilled water
- Flush cannulated instruments with distilled water followed by forced air from a syringe
- Sterilize instruments according to manufacturer recommendations

Microkeratome

- Swab motor handpiece with ethanol
- Advance and reverse motor tip while dipped in ethanol or acetone to remove debris
- Avoid blade reuse

Sterilizer

- Evacuate sterilizer water reservoir and dry thoroughly one to two times per week (see Figure 5)
- Use Pyrogen-free sterile water for the sterilizer

Host Factors

- Treat blepharitis preoperatively
- Treat atopic patients and patients with a prior history of DLK with prednisone 60 mg po qid starting 1 day prior to surgery

Intraoperative Precautions

- Use a betadine prep and drape eyelids
- Use an aspirating lid speculum or a sponge to minimize fluid reflux into flap interface
- Complete a thorough washout of the interface if any debris is noted
- Avoid epithelial defects by using viscous ocular lubricants (Celluvisc/Cellufresh) intraoperatively

loss, as the stroma is quite soft resulting in a significant hyperopic shift and irregular astigmatism. These complications may slowly improve over the next 3 to 6 months. In addition, patients with resultant scarring may slowly return to their preoperative BCVA over the next 6 to 12 months.[10] We suggest waiting at least this long before considering topography or wavefront guided customized corneal ablation when these modalities become readily available.

Prevention

Since the etiology for any given case of DLK is likely multifactorial, the prevention of this entity is also multifactorial (Table 4). When multiple cases occur at the same center on 1 day, then attention may be focused to prevent further contamination with potential bacterial byproducts (endotoxins[11] and exotoxins). Special attention should be paid to the proper cleaning and drying of the sterilizing equipment (Figure 5). Holland, Shumer, and others have advocated draining the sterilizer's reservoir at least one to two times per week to avoid contamination

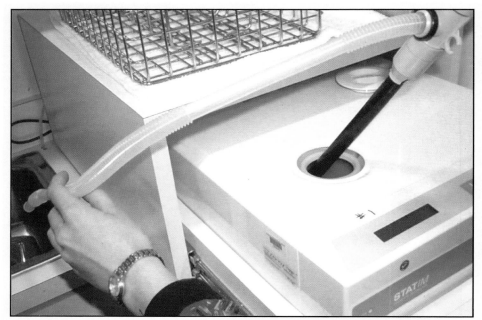

Figure 5. The sterilizer water reservoir should be evacuated and dried thoroughly one to two times per week to avoid bacterial accumulation in the water reservoir. The sterilizer inactivates the bacteria, but the cellular byproducts (endotoxins) can cause inflammation.

with bacterial byproducts. The use of pyrogen free sterile water in the sterilizer is also indicated. In addition, meticulous attention to the cleaning of all instruments and the microkeratome is recommended.

Peters, et al performed a prospective study of the application of prednisolone sodium phosphate 1% on the undersurface of the flap immediately after it was reflected during LASIK.[12] The incidence of DLK in treated eyes was 6.7% versus 17.1% of the untreated eyes, however the observers were not masked to the treatment versus control groups. Both the steroid and the control groups had a greater incidence of interface keratitis than previously reported and this is likely attributed to more meticulous and frequent postoperative examinations and the criteria used for making the diagnosis.

Conclusions

DLK is a vision-threatening problem that must be recognized and treated immediately. Once identified, stage 1 and 2 should be treated with hourly high potency topical steroids, with close follow-up in 24 to 48 hours. If BCVA is decreased more than one to two lines and clumping of cells occurs in the visual axis, then the addition of high dose oral corticosteroids (prednisone 60 to 80 mg/day) and immediate lifting of the flap with copious irrigation is essential. As more knowledge is obtained about the potential etiologies of DLK, better modalities may be developed to prevent its occurrence. Until then, the focus must be on the accurate and early diagnosis of the disorder followed by aggressive and definitive treatment.

References

1.   Maddox R, Hatsis A. Shifting Sands of the Sahara: Interface inflammation following LASIK. In: Gimbel HV, Anderson Penno EE, eds. *LASIK Complications: Prevention and Management*. Thorofare, NJ: SLACK Incorporated; 1999:30-36.

2.   Smith RJ, Maloney RK. Diffuse lamellar keratitis: A new syndrome in lamellar refractive surgery. *Ophthalmology*. 1998;105:1721-1726.

3.   Moyer PD, Khanna R, Berbos TG, et al. Interface keratitis after LASIK may be caused by microkeratome lubricant deposits. *Invest Ophthalmol Vis Sci*. 1998;39(suppl):S750.

4.   Kaufman SC, Maitchouk DY, Chiou AG, Beuerman RW. Interface inflammation after laser in situ keratomileusis-Sands of the Sahara syndrome. *J Cataract Refract Surg*. 1998;24:1589-1593.

5.   Macaluso DC, Rich LF, MacRae, SM. Sterile interface keratitis after laser in situ keratomileusis: Three episodes in one patient with concomitant contact dermatitis of the eyelids. *J Refract Surg*. 1999;15:679-682.

6.   MacRae SM, Macaluso DC, Rich LF. Sterile interface keratitis associated with micropannus hemorrhage after laser in situ keratomileusis. *J Cataract Refract Surg*. 1999;25(12):1679-1681.

7.   Machat JJ. LASIK complications. In: Machat JJ, Slade SG, Probst LE, eds. *The Art of LASIK, Second Edition*. Thorofare, NJ: SLACK Incorporated; 1999:392-396.

8.   Linebarger EJ, Hardten DR, Lindstrom RL. Sands of the Sahara. In: Buratto L, Brint S, eds. *LASIK: Surgical Techniques and Complications*. Thorofare, NJ: SLACK Incorporated; 2000:591-596.

9.   MacRae, SM, Rich LF. The use of oral corticosteroids to control inflammation and interface keratitis after LASIK (ARVO abstract). *Invest Ophthalmol Vis Sci*. (Abstract 1680). 2000;41(40:S318..

10. Fraenkel GE, Cohen PR, Sutton GL, Lawless MA, Rogers CM. Central focal interface opacity after laser in situ keratomileusis. *J Refract Surg*. 1998;14:571-576.

11. Doane JF. Diffuse interlamellar keratitis: Sands of the Sahara syndrome. In: Buratto L, Brint S, eds. *LASIK: Surgical Techniques and Complications*. Thorofare, NJ: SLACK Incorporated; 2000:581-588.

12. Peters NT, Lingua RW, Kim CH. Topical intrastromal steroid during laser in situ keratomileusis to retard interface keratitis. *J Cataract Refract Surg*. 1999;25:1437-1440.

REFERENCES

1.   Gimbel HV, Iskander NG, Peters NT, Anderson Penno EE. Prevention and management of microkeratome-related LASIK complications. *J Cataract Refract Surg*. 2000;16(2):S226-229.

2.   Iskander NG, Peters NT, Anderson Penno EE, Gimbel, HV. *Postoperative complications in LASIK, Current Opinion in Ophthalmology*. 2000;11(4): 273-279.

3.   Kim HM, Song JK, Han HS, Jung HR. Streptococcal keratitis after myopic laser in situ keratomileusis. *Korean J Ophthalmol*. 1998;12:108-111.

4.   Webber SK, Lawless MA, Sutton GL, Rogers CM. Staphylococcal infection under a LASIK flap. *Cornea*. 1999;18(3):361-365.

5. Perez-Santonja JJ, Sakla HF, Abad JL, Zarraquino A, Esteban J, Alio JL. Nocardial keratitis after laser in situ keratomileusis. *J Refract Surg.* 1997;13:314-317.

6. Haw WW, Manche EE. Sterile peripheral keratitis following laser in situ keratomileusis. *J Refract Surg.* 1999;15:61-63.

7. Lam DS, Leung AT, Wu JT, Fan DS, Cheng AC, Wang Z. Culture-negative ulcerative keratitis after laser in situ keratomileusis. *J Refract Surg.* 1999;25:1004-1008.

8. Aras C, Ozdamar A, Bahcecioglu, H, Bozkurt S. Corneal interface abscess after excimer laser in situ keratomileusis. *J Refract Surg.* 1998;14:156-157.

9. Davidorf JM. Herpes simplex keratitis after LASIK. Letter to the editor. *J Refract Surg.* 1998;14:667.

10. Smith RJ, Maloney RK. Diffuse lamellar keratitis. A new syndrome in lamellar refractive surgery. *Ophthalmology.* 1998;105:1721-1726.

11. Kaufman SC, Maitchouk DY, Chiou AG, Beuerman RW. Interface inflammation after laser in situ keratomileusis, Sands of Sahara syndrome. *J Cataract Refract Surg.* 1998; 24:1589-1593.

12. Lineberger EJ, Hardten DR, Chu RY, Lindstrom RL. Understanding time course of DLK can eliminate visual loss. *Ocular Surgery News.* Sept 1, 1999;17(17):11-12.

13. Kaufman SC, Maitchouk DY, Chiou AG, Beuerman RW. Post LASIK interface keratitis, Sands of Sahara syndrome, and microkeratome blades. Letter to the editor. *J Cataract Refract Surg.* 1999; 25:603-604.

14. Maloney RK. Sterile interface inflammation after laser in situ keratomileusis: Experience and opinions. *J Refract Surg.* 1998;14:661.

15. Peters NT, Lingua RW, Kim CH. Topical intrastromal steroid during laser in situ keratomileusis to retard interface inflammation. *J Cataract Refract Surg.* 1999;25:1437-1440.

16. Hirst LW, Vandeleur KW. Laser in situ keratomileusis interface deposits. *J Refract Surg.* 1998;14:653-654.

17. Campos M, Carvalho MJ, Scarpi M, Chamon W. Excimer laser intrastromal keratomileusis (LASIK): A clinical follow-up. *Ophthalmic Surgery and Lasers.* 1996(suppl);27(5):S534.

18. Maloney RK. Epithelial ingrowth after lamellar refractive surgery. *Ophthalmic Surgery and Lasers.* 1996(suppl);27(5):S535.

19. Wilson SE. LASIK Complications. *Cornea.* 1998;17(5):459-467.

20. Gimbel HV, Peters NT, Iskander NG, Anderson Penno EE. LASIK flap complications and management. *J Refract Surg.* 2000;16(2):S223-225.

21. Gimbel HV, Levy SG. Indications, results and complications of LASIK. *Current Opinion in Ophthalmology.* 1998;9(IV):3-8.

22. Gimbel HV, Anderson Penno EE, van Westenbrugge JA, Ferensowicz M, Furlong MT. Incidence and management of intra and early postoperative complications in 1000 consecutive LASIK cases. *Ophthalmology.* 1998;105:1839-1848.

23. Stulting RD, Carr JD, Thompson KP, Waring GO, Wiley WM, Walker JG. Complications of laser in situ keratomileusis for the correction of myopia. *Ophthalmology.* 1999;106:13-20.

24. Lamm DSC, Leung ATS, Wu JT, et al. Management of severe flap wrinkling or dislodgment after laser in situ keratomileusis. *J Cataract Refract Surg.* 1999;25(11):1441-1447.

7

Late Postoperative Complications

Several complications may present after the first 24 to 48 hours. These late complications may require additional surgical intervention, and patients should be advised to seek prompt evaluation from their eye care provider if they experience increasing blurred vision or discomfort.

EPITHELIAL INGROWTH

Epithelial ingrowth is usually noted within the first few weeks after surgery (Figure 7-1). It most commonly occurs after enhancement surgery and after a flap complication.[1-3] Stulting, et al reported a 1.5% incidence of epithelial ingrowth.[4] In our first 1000 patients, we have reported a 3.5% incidence of epithelial ingrowth.[5] The majority of these cases are quite mild at the edge of the flap and do not require treatment. The epithelial cells may have a limited proliferative potential. If so, a nest of cells may appear, stop expanding, and remain stable for years. Occasionally, they will continue to grow and may produce significant complications.[6] The slit lamp appearance of epithelial ingrowth may vary (Figures 7-1, 7-2a and b). It may appear as a peninsula extending from the flap edge with a whorl pattern, or as a gray, necrotic appearance to the flap edge resulting in a stromal melt. In some cases small cysts or pearls of epithelium occur at the flap

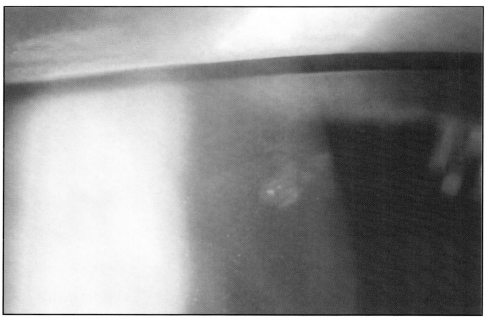

Figure 7-1. High magnification of a small area of epithelial ingrowth. (Reprinted with permission from Gimbel HV, Anderson Penno EE. *LASIK Complications: Prevention and Management.* Thorofare, NJ: SLACK Incorporated, 1999.)

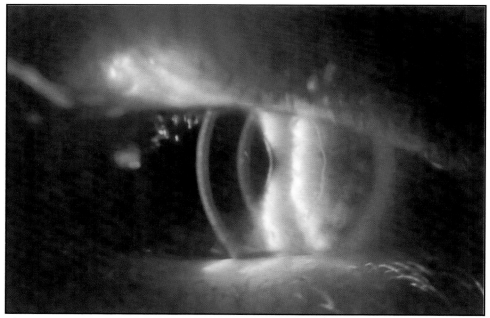

Figure 7-2a. A variety of appearances can be found in cases of epithelial ingrowth (see Patient Example 22). (Reprinted with permission from Gimbel HV, Anderson Penno EE. *LASIK Complications: Prevention and Management.* Thorofare, NJ: SLACK Incorporated, 1999.)

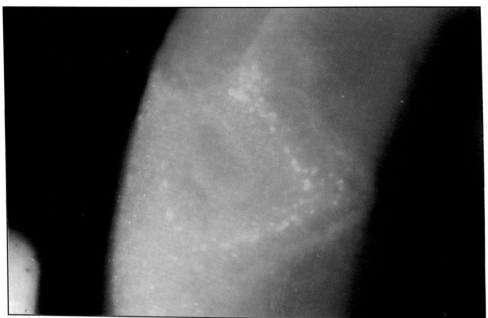

Figure 7-2b. This patient underwent debridement and recovered uncorrected visual acuity of 20/15[-1] at 6 weeks post-debridement (see Patient Example 22). (Reprinted with permission from Gimbel HV, Anderson Penno EE. *LASIK Complications: Prevention and Management.* Thorofare, NJ: SLACK Incorporated, 1999.)

edge. Irregular astigmatism affecting the corneal maps and refraction may result from the ingrowth extending centrally. The visual acuity may be decreased. Patients may also complain of irritation or pain related to irregularities of the corneal surface.

Risk factors include poor flap adhesion, epithelial abrasions involving the flap edge, flap misalignment, and buttonholes (Table 7-1). Hyperopic LASIK should not be done with the 9 mm transition zone unless the flap edge is outside the margins of the ablation because there is a higher risk of epithelial ingrowth when the ablation affects the edge of the flap cut, especially at the hinge end.[7] The rates of epithelial ingrowth following hyperopic LASIK have been reported to be as high as 31.4%.[8] The risk for epithelial ingrowth may also be greater following retreatments due to irregularities and tags that may be present following dissection of the flap. To minimize this risk, the edges of the stromal bed must be meticulously cleaned of any epithelial tags or debris prior to repositioning the flap.

The hallmark of management is prevention (see Table 7-1). Flaps with progressive enlargement of epithelial ingrowth should be gently lifted and the edges carefully cleared of epithelium with a Paton spatula. The epithelium on the bed and the underside of the flap should be scraped, while maintaining the flap integrity.[3]

Some surgeons advocate using minimal laser spots or 50% *alcohol solution* on the stromal bed and the underlying surface of the cap to prevent recurrences. Debridement of both the stromal surface and the undersurface of the flap shoul

Table 7-1

Epithelial Ingrowth

Possible Causes	• Poor flap edge adhesion • Epithelial abrasions at the flap edge • Flap misalignment • Buttonholes • Spillover of ablation at the bed margins • Irregularities or epithelial tags at the bed margins on enhancements
Results	• Decreased visual acuity • Irregular astigmatism • Discomfort (relating to surface irregularities) • Risk of stromal melt
Solutions	*Avoidance* • Meticulous attention to epithelium on primary and enhancement surgeries • Carefully approximate all torn epithelium at edges of the flap • Clear any epithelium, tags, or debris from stromal bed prior to flap repositioning • Avoid large transition zones on small beds and shield hinge area as necessary *Management* • Very small area at flap edge with vision changes can be monitored carefully • Visually significant ingrowth or an area of epithelial ingrowth >1 to 2 mm requires treatment • Lift the flap after clearing edges of epithelial tags or debris with the Paton spatula • Debride the stromal surface and undersurface of flap edges using a clean sponge for each pass

(Reprinted with permission from Gimbel HV, Anderson Penno EE. LASIK Complications: Prevention and Management. Thorofare, NJ: SLACK Incorporated, 1999.)

performed using the Paton spatula.[3,7,10] All epithelial tags should be meticulously cleaned from the edge of the stromal bed using the Paton spatula prior to repositioning of the flap.

STROMAL MELTS

...sis, or melting of the flap, is a serious complication. It may be caused by ...rowth in the interface (Figure 7-3).[7] It has also been reported follow-...flammatory interface debris.[7] In our experience, this has been a rare ...wever some authors have reported an incidence as high as 5.7%.[11] ...e etiology of keratolysis is unknown. It has been proposed that ...vation of the flap stroma from its essential nutrient, glucose.[9] ...th acts as a mechanical barrier in the interface between the ...ueous humor from the anterior chamber rich in glucose.[9]

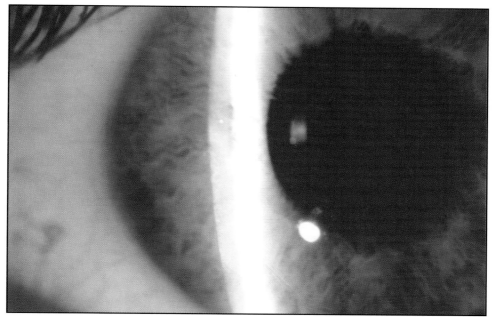

Figure 7-3. Loss of stroma in the flap "melt" caused by epithelial ingrowth.

This may result in necrosis of the flap stromal tissue. Inflammatory etiologies mediated by cytokines have also been proposed.[12] Prevention of keratolysis involves early recognition and prompt treatment of any inflammatory process or epithelial ingrowth.

OVERCORRECTION/UNDERCORRECTION

Simple overcorrection and undercorrection will be apparent within the first week. Overcorrections are more common following LASIK as compared to PRK.[6] The refraction and map contours following LASIK for low and moderate myopia have been reported to stabilize as early as 3 months postoperatively.[13] Enhancements for undercorrection or overcorrection following primary LASIK for myopia or hyperopia can be performed as early as 3 to 6 months after the primary procedure. The refraction should be stable, as demonstrated by similar refractions one month apart. The flap can be easily lifted and simple blunt dissection is performed up to a year or later after the primary procedure followed by retreatment of the stromal bed. We (and others) have lifted the flap in this manner as long as 3 years after primary myopic LASIK.[7,14] Occasionally, an adherent flap is encountered if the cut or the ablation left a rough surface and more than usual fibrosis occurred in the healing process, or if the flap edge is quite near the limbus. These flap edges can be replaced and a recut done in 2 to 3 months. The flaps tend to be more adherent to the stromal bed following hyperopic LASIK. We recommend recutting of the flap for enhancement after 12 months following hyperopic LASIK if the previous ablation was near the edge of the flap. If a large flap was used it may be lifted as easily as after myopic LASIK.[7]

The best way to avoid unnecessary enhancements for simple undercorrections or overcorrections is to obtain accurate preoperative measurements, including cycloplegic refraction, and to adopt a method of continuous improvement with regard to laser treatment algorithms. Examples of algorithms are shown in Tables 7-2a through c, as well as in Chapter 3. These algorithms are heavily dependent on laser type and may also be affected by intraoperative technique (most likely related to tissue hydration status), laser suite conditions (such as ambient humidity and temperature), and geographic location of the laser center. Some studies indicate that patient age may also be important.[15]

Algorithms also differ from LASIK as compared to PRK due to the difference in ablation rates of Bowman's membrane and stroma; this difference may also be related to hydration status or techniques of epithelial removal in PRK (eg, the use of ethanol as an epithelial softening agent).

Algorithms for hyperopic LASIK and astigmatic corrections lag behind simple myopic corrections. However, as experience is gained, these algorithms are becoming more accurate. Furthermore, inaccuracy in algorithms will make a larger difference in higher attempted corrections. For example, a 10% error in a 2.0 D correction is quite insignificant while a 10% error in a 12.0 D correction will be visually significant. A larger response can be expected on retreatments of overcorrections, especially in hyperopic treatments for overcorrected myopia. Therefore, the algorithms used for retreatments should be quite different than those used for primary LASIK. We use 50% of the correction used in primary LASIK.

We recommend that computerized records and a database be kept with regard to all patients and a periodic review be made to evaluate the attempted versus achieved laser corrections. Modifications in techniques and software must also be taken into consideration when reviewing these data. This policy of continuous improvement is an iterative process that results in increasing accuracy in corrections. In addition, a system of double checks is built into our routine for entering the corrections into the laser, such that the numbers, the correct eye, the correct axis verified by looking at a topographical map, and the correct patient are verified by a second person and the surgeon to avoid typographical or entry errors.

The specifics of surgical techniques involved in lifting the flap for LASIK retreatments will be discussed in detail in Chapter 8.

Regression

Regression is less common following LASIK as compared to following PRK, possibly because the Bowman's membrane is preserved in LASIK.[3,6] Preoperative high myopia is more likely to regress than low to moderate myopia. Hyperopia and high astigmatism are also more prone to regression following primary LASIK treatment. Enhancements should be delayed until the refractions are stable. There is no evidence that the use of prophylactic steroids carries any benefit in the avoidance of regression following LASIK.

Table 7-2a and b

Nidek PRK and LASIK Algorithms

(a)

Optical Zone (mm)	PRK (%)	LASIK (%)
5.5–7.0	78	86
6.0–7.0	76	86
6.5–7.0	74	84
6.5–7.5	72	82

(b)

Optical Zone (mm)	*PRK (%)	LASIK (%)
5.5–7.0	78	84
6.0–7.0	78	82
6.5–7.0	74	80
6.5–7.5	72	78

* For patients > 35 years old, these numbers are decreased by 3%.

These tables are examples of how algorithms are used at two different centers for myopia treatment. Not only do the algorithms differ for PRK versus LASIK, but they also differ between centers. Each center will have its own algorithms based on a variety of factors.

(Reprinted with permission from Gimbel HV, Anderson Penno EE. LASIK Complications: Prevention and Management. *Thorofare, NJ: SLACK Incorporated, 1999.)*

Table 7-2c

Positive Effect of Minus Cylinder Correction on Sphere Using Nidek EC-5000

Preop Cyl (D)	%	Effect (D)
−0.50	0.35	+0.175
−0.75	0.35	+0.263
−1.00	0.35	+0.350
−1.25	0.35	+0.438
−1.50	0.35	+0.525
−1.75	0.35	+0.613
−2.00	0.35	+0.700
−2.25	0.35	+0.788
−2.50	0.35	+0.875
−2.75	0.35	+0.963
−3.00	0.35	+0.963
−3.00	0.35	+1.050
−3.25	0.35	+1.138
−3.50	0.35	+1.225
−3.75	0.35	+1.313
−4.00	0.35	+1.400
−4.25	0.35	+1.488
−4.50	0.35	+1.575

Table 7-2c continued		
Preop Cyl (D)	**%**	**Effect (D)**
–4.75	0.35	+1.663
–5.00	0.35	+1.750
–5.25	0.35	+1.838
–5.50	0.35	+1.838
–5.50	0.35	+1.925
–5.75	0.35	+2.013
–6.00	0.35	+2.100
–6.25	0.35	+2.188
–6.50	0.25	+2.275
–6.75	0.35	+2.363
–7.00	0.35	+2.450

(Reprinted with permission from Gimbel HV, Anderson Penno EE. LASIK Complications: Prevention and Management. Thorofare, NJ: SLACK Incorporated, 1999.)

HAZE

Haze is also less common following LASIK as compared to following PRK, and occurs only rarely. Epithelial ingrowth or interface debris should be ruled out in the differential diagnosis. Interface haze may be due to the toxins in the intra-operative fluids used. Interface haze has been reported to respond to topical steroids.[16] A pattern of crystalline haze can be seen following hyperopic ablations (Figure 7-4). This is usually not visually significant and does not require steroid therapy. It can be minimized by performing a final PTK smoothing using a special smoothing fluid just after treatment.[7]

CENTRAL ISLANDS

The primary cause of central islands after LASIK appears to be the profile of the delivery beam and the older software in broadbeam laser systems. Central islands may be the most common topographical abnormality following LASIK treatment using a broadbeam laser.[17] Central islands have become much less common with newer software modifications and are seen only rarely after treatment with scanning slit and flying spot lasers. Uneven stromal hydration or obstruction to laser energy from the plume of ejected corneal vapor may also play a role in the formation of central islands.

Patients may present with glare, ghosting, and undercorrections. Corneal topography will reveal an island, isthmus, or peninsula pattern. There is little tendency for central islands to resolve following LASIK as compared to PRK.[6] If persistent, PTK smoothing can be performed on the stromal bed under the flap. A hyperopic shift may result from removal of central tissue during retreatment, therefore a conservative approach is warranted when treating central islands.

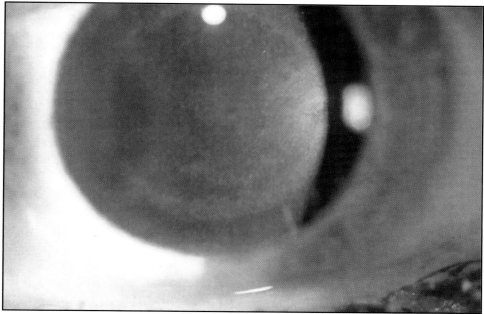

Figure 7-4. Annular haze after hyperopic LASIK. (Reprinted with permission from Gimbel HV, Anderson Penno EE. *LASIK Complications: Prevention and Management.* Thorofare, NJ: SLACK Incorporated, 1999.)

Table 7-3
Causes of Irregular Astigmatism
•Wrinkles or folds in the flap •Interface debris •Epithelial ingrowth •Decentration
(Reprinted with permission from Gimbel HV, Anderson Penno EE. LASIK Complications: Prevention and Management. Thorofare, NJ: SLACK Incorporated, 1999.)

IRREGULAR ASTIGMATISM

Wrinkles or folds in the flap are the most common cause of irregular astigmatism. It can also be caused by flap misalignment, central island, debris or epithelial ingrowth in the stromal-flap interface, and decentration of the ablation (Table 7-3). Irregular astigmatism can be a major cause of lost BCVA or visual disturbances. Waring, et al reported a 3.3% loss of two or more lines at 1 year, secondary to irregular astigmatism.[18] Retreatments in these cases should be directed by the underlying causes. If caused by wrinkles and detected early, the flap should be refloated and smoothed. If detected later, a surface PTK smoothing can be performed, or the flap can be lifted and massaged with a dry sponge or blunt instrument to stretch out the wrinkles.[19]

SMALL OPTICAL ZONE

The advent of newer lasers employing larger optical zones has markedly decreased this problem.[7] Patients with large scotopic pupils and higher corrections are at a higher risk for night vision effects of halos and glare. Patients with thin corneas and/or large corrections will be limited to a small optical zone to respect the 250 μ bed that should remain due to the theoretic risk of keratectasia. Patients with these parameters should be counseled regarding their suitability for LASIK and may need to be referred for an alternative procedure such as lensectomy or phakic IOL.[7] If the cornea is thick enough, the optical zone may be enlarged by various methods (including placing a hyperopic correction followed immediately by a wide diameter myopic ablation).[20]

DECENTRATION

Decentration may present with loss of BCVA, irregular astigmatism, and visual aberrations such as ghosting and night vision disturbances. Decentration may be primarily caused by poor fixation as a result of poor patient instruction, patient agitation, loss of concentration secondary to heavy sedation, or blurred vision resulting from high refractive errors or difficulty seeing through the exposed stromal bed. Iatrogenic decentration can occur with improper use of the Thornton ring (see Figure 5-21). Secondary decentration may be an artifact of uneven healing with patchy haze formation.[3]

Mild degrees of decentration can be treated with a small diameter (3 to 4 mm) ablation at the edge of the original optical zone decentered in an opposite direction, thus enlarging the optical zone in the pupillary axis (Figures 7-5a and b). A hyperopic shift may occur due to the removal of tissue centrally by this method. This method is difficult to use following LASIK, as retreatment will be constrained by the size of the bed. Special care must be taken not to ablate over the edges of the bed, as this may pose a risk for epithelial ingrowth. Other approaches include placement of a retreatment centered on the pupil and rely on the flap to smooth the combined treatment zone or using arcuate incisions placed just outside the flap edge at the steep corneal axis.[14,20] Custom ablations or topography-guided laser ablations (TopoLink) may provide a future hope for treatment of decentration (see Chapter 3).[7]

Retreatment for decentration may be difficult, ineffective, and limited by the flap diameter—regardless of the method used. It may be possible in difficult cases to use the epithelium as a template such that the proposed treatment is placed onto the epithelium with care to avoid breakthrough to the stroma (Figure 7-6). Topography can be performed immediately following treatment and if the pattern is centered, the epithelium can then be allowed to heal prior to performing the same treatment on the stromal bed. In these cases, the patient must be advised that more than one retreatment may be required.

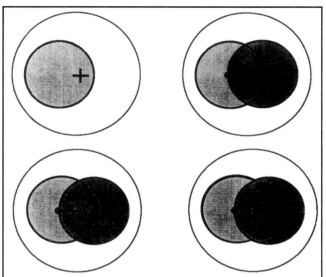

Figure 7-5a. Decentration. For mild degrees of decentration, a small diameter ablation may be performed at the edge of the original optical zone to enlarge the optical zone in the pupillary axis. (Reprinted with permission from Gimbel HV, Anderson Penno EE. *LASIK Complications: Prevention and Management.* Thorofare, NJ: SLACK Incorporated, 1999.)

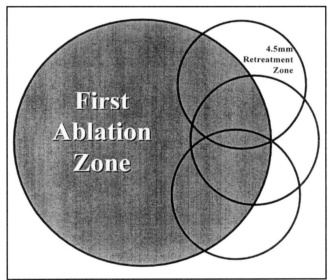

Figure 7-5b. Decentration. A series of three small diameter ablations may be placed at the edge of the decentered ablation followed by PTK smoothing. (Reprinted with permission from Gimbel HV, Anderson Penno EE. *LASIK Complications: Prevention and Management.* Thorofare, NJ: SLACK Incorporated, 1999.)

Figure 7-6. A pattern can be imprinted on the epithelium with topography to be performed immediately postoperatively. Care needs to be taken not to break through to stroma during the initial treatment. If the topography is satisfactory, the patient can be allowed to heal prior to performing the same treatment on the stromal bed. (Reprinted with permission from Gimbel HV, Anderson Penno EE. *LASIK Complications: Prevention and Management.* Thorofare, NJ: SLACK Incorporated, 1999.)

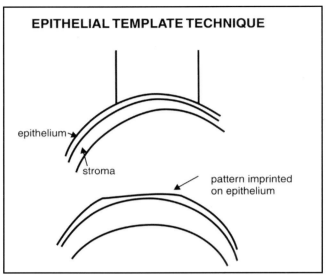

KERATECTASIA

The consensus among LASIK surgeons is that at least 250 μ should remain in the stromal bed following laser ablation.[21-25] However, in a retrospective analysis of 2000 consecutive myopic LASIK eyes we did not find a correlation between total residual bed thickness and latest spherical equivalent (Presented at the AAO 1999 Annual Meeting in Orlando. Postoperative corneal thinning masquerading as undercorrection or regression in LASIK Surgery.). The majority of reports of iatrogenic keratectasia following LASIK found less than 200μ bed was left after ablation or in cases of a forme fruste keratoconus; but there have also been cases in which >250 μ bed thickness remained.[21-24] Excessive thinning of the stromal bed may theoretically lead to biomechanical weakening of the cornea, causing a posterior keratoconus, which may manifest months after the procedure.[22,25] Some surgeons have proposed that keratectasia is due to the action of the IOP on the weakened cornea.[23]

The timing of the development of keratectasia is not clear, although it has been reported in the literature to develop between 1 and 9 months following surgery.[21-22,24,26-27] Corneal topography reveals progressive steepening at the site of the pathology (Figures 7-7a, b, and c). The steepening appears to be more pronounced in older patients.[28] Management of keratectasia is difficult. Conservative management with rigid gas permeable contact lenses is the first line of management.[21] In severe cases with loss of BCVA, an epikeratoplasty or a penetrating keratoplasty may be the only alternative.[7,21] In high corrections limited by pupil size and corneal thickness, techniques of combined sequential refractive surgery may be used to limit the disadvantages of each technique.[7]

The hallmark of the management of keratectasia is prevention. Residual corneal bed thickness can be calculated using the Munnerlyn formula (Figures 7-8a, b, and c). Patients who present with keratoconus or form fruste keratoconus may be at high risk for keratectasia following LASIK.

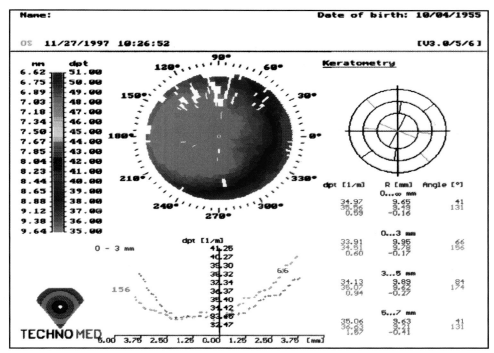

Figure 7-7a. Progressive steepening resulting from krectasia can be seen on corneal mapping.

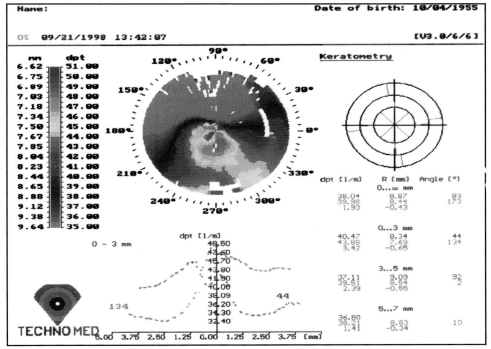

Figure 7-7b. Progressive steepening resulting from krectasia can be seen on corneal mapping.

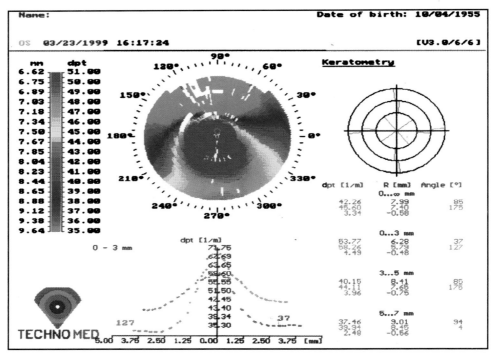

Figure 7-7c. Progressive steepening resulting from krectasia can be seen on corneal mapping.

Figure 7-8a. Munnerlyn formula, ablation depth, and optical zone calculation. (Reprinted with permission from Gimbel HV, Anderson Penno EE. *LASIK Complications: Prevention and Management.* Thorofare, NJ: SLACK Incorporated, 1999.)

Munnerlyn Formula

$$T = (Dh^2)/3$$

T = Thickness in microns
D = Power in diopters
h = Diameter of optical zone in millimeters

Ablation Depth (υm)

Diopters	Optical Zone									
	3	3.5	4	4.5	5	5.5	6	6.5	7	7.5
0.50	1.50	2.04	2.67	3.38	4.17	5.04	6.00	7.04	8.17	9.38
0.75	2.25	3.06	4.00	5.06	6.25	7.56	9.00	10.56	12.25	14.06
1.00	3.00	4.08	5.33	6.75	8.33	10.08	12.00	14.08	16.33	18.75
1.25	3.75	5.10	6.67	8.44	10.42	12.60	15.00	17.60	20.42	23.44
1.50	4.50	6.13	8.00	10.13	12.50	15.13	18.00	21.13	24.50	28.13
1.75	5.25	7.15	9.33	11.81	14.58	17.65	21.00	24.65	28.58	32.81
2.00	6.00	8.17	10.67	13.50	16.67	20.17	24.00	28.17	32.67	37.50
2.25	6.75	9.19	12.00	15.19	18.75	22.69	27.00	31.69	36.75	42.19
2.50	7.50	10.21	13.33	16.88	20.83	25.21	30.00	35.21	40.83	46.88
2.75	8.25	11.23	14.67	18.56	22.92	27.73	33.00	38.73	44.92	51.56
3.00	9.00	12.25	16.00	20.25	25.00	30.25	36.00	42.25	49.00	56.25
3.25	9.75	13.27	17.33	21.94	27.08	32.77	39.00	45.77	53.08	60.94
3.50	10.50	14.29	18.67	23.63	29.17	35.29	42.00	49.29	57.17	65.63
3.75	11.25	15.31	20.00	25.31	31.25	37.81	45.00	52.81	61.25	70.31
4.00	12.00	16.33	21.33	27.00	33.33	40.33	48.00	56.33	65.33	75.00
4.25	12.75	17.35	22.67	28.69	35.42	42.85	51.00	59.85	69.42	79.69
4.50	13.50	18.38	24.00	30.38	37.50	45.38	54.00	63.38	73.50	84.38
4.75	14.25	19.40	25.33	32.06	39.58	47.90	57.00	66.90	77.58	89.06
5.00	15.00	20.42	26.67	33.75	41.67	50.42	60.00	70.42	81.67	93.75
5.25	15.75	21.44	28.00	35.44	43.75	52.94	63.00	73.94	85.75	98.44
5.50	16.50	22.46	29.33	37.13	45.83	55.46	66.00	77.46	89.83	103.13
5.75	17.25	23.48	30.67	38.81	47.92	57.98	69.00	80.98	93.92	107.81
6.00	18.00	24.50	32.00	40.50	50.00	60.50	72.00	84.50	98.00	112.50
6.25	18.75	25.52	33.33	42.19	52.08	63.02	75.00	88.02	102.08	117.19
6.50	19.50	26.54	34.67	43.88	54.17	65.54	78.00	91.54	106.17	121.88
6.75	20.25	27.56	36.00	45.56	56.25	68.06	81.00	95.06	110.25	126.56
7.00	21.00	28.58	37.33	47.25	58.33	70.58	84.00	98.58	114.33	131.25
7.25	21.75	29.60	38.67	48.94	60.42	73.10	87.00	102.10	118.42	135.94
7.50	22.50	30.63	40.00	50.63	62.50	75.63	90.00	105.63	122.50	140.63
7.75	23.25	31.65	41.33	52.31	64.58	78.15	93.00	109.15	126.58	145.31
8.00	24.00	32.67	42.67	54.00	66.67	80.67	96.00	112.67	130.67	150.00
8.25	24.75	33.69	44.00	55.69	68.75	83.19	99.00	116.19	134.75	154.69
8.50	25.50	34.71	45.33	57.38	70.83	85.71	102.00	119.71	138.83	159.38
8.75	26.25	35.73	46.67	59.06	72.92	88.23	105.00	123.23	142.92	164.06
9.00	27.00	36.75	48.00	60.75	75.00	90.75	108.00	126.75	147.00	168.75
9.25	27.75	37.77	49.33	62.44	77.08	93.27	111.00	130.27	151.08	173.44
9.50	28.50	38.79	50.67	64.13	79.17	95.79	114.00	133.79	155.17	178.13
9.75	29.25	39.81	52.00	65.81	81.25	98.31	117.00	137.31	159.25	182.81
10.00	30.00	40.83	53.33	67.50	83.33	100.83	120.00	140.83	163.33	187.50

Figure 7-8b. Using the Munnerlyn formula, an ablation depth chart was created. One can also calculate the ablation depth for a given optical zone and treatment. For example, a 4.50 D treatment in a 3 mm zone gets an ablation depth of 13.5 μ, and a 10.00 D ablation with an optical zone of 7.5 mm would require an ablation depth of 187.5 μ. (Reprinted with permission from Gimbel HV, Anderson Penno EE. *LASIK Complications: Prevention and Management.* Thorofare, NJ: SLACK Incorporated, 1999.)

Optical Zone Calculation (250um)

Corneal Thickness (T)

Diopters:	430	440	450	460	470	480	490	500	510	520	530	540	550	560	570	580	590	600	610
1.00	7.75	9.49	10.95	12.25	13.42	14.49	15.49	16.43	17.32	18.17	18.97	19.75	20.49	21.21	21.91	22.58	23.24	23.87	24.49
1.50	6.32	7.75	8.94	10.00	10.95	11.83	12.65	13.42	14.14	14.83	15.49	16.12	16.73	17.32	17.89	18.44	18.97	19.49	20.00
2.00	5.48	6.71	7.75	8.66	9.49	10.25	10.95	11.62	12.25	12.85	13.42	13.96	14.49	15.00	15.49	15.97	16.43	16.88	17.32
2.50	4.90	6.00	6.93	7.75	8.49	9.17	9.80	10.39	10.95	11.49	12.00	12.49	12.96	13.42	13.86	14.28	14.70	15.10	15.49
3.00	4.47	5.48	6.32	7.07	7.75	8.37	8.94	9.49	10.00	10.49	10.95	11.40	11.83	12.25	12.65	13.04	13.42	13.78	14.14
3.50	4.14	5.07	5.86	6.55	7.17	7.75	8.28	8.78	9.26	9.71	10.14	10.56	10.95	11.34	11.71	12.07	12.42	12.76	13.09
4.00	3.87	4.74	5.48	6.12	6.71	7.25	7.75	8.22	8.66	9.08	9.49	9.87	10.25	10.61	10.95	11.29	11.62	11.94	12.25
4.50	3.65	4.47	5.16	5.77	6.32	6.83	7.30	7.75	8.16	8.56	8.94	9.31	9.66	10.00	10.33	10.65	10.95	11.25	11.55
5.00	3.46	4.24	4.90	5.48	6.00	6.48	6.93	7.35	7.75	8.12	8.49	8.83	9.17	9.49	9.80	10.10	10.39	10.68	10.95
5.50	3.30	4.05	4.67	5.22	5.72	6.18	6.61	7.01	7.39	7.75	8.09	8.42	8.74	9.05	9.34	9.63	9.91	10.18	10.44
6.00	3.16	3.87	4.47	5.00	5.48	5.92	6.32	6.71	7.07	7.42	7.75	8.06	8.37	8.66	8.94	9.22	9.49	9.75	10.00
6.50	3.04	3.72	4.30	4.80	5.26	5.68	6.08	6.45	6.79	7.13	7.44	7.75	8.04	8.32	8.59	8.86	9.11	9.36	9.61
7.00	2.93	3.59	4.14	4.63	5.07	5.48	5.86	6.21	6.55	6.87	7.17	7.46	7.75	8.02	8.28	8.54	8.78	9.02	9.26
7.50	2.83	3.46	4.00	4.47	4.90	5.29	5.66	6.00	6.32	6.63	6.93	7.21	7.48	7.75	8.00	8.25	8.49	8.72	8.94
8.00	2.74	3.35	3.87	4.33	4.74	5.12	5.48	5.81	6.12	6.42	6.71	6.98	7.25	7.50	7.75	7.98	8.22	8.44	8.66
8.50	2.66	3.25	3.76	4.20	4.60	4.97	5.31	5.64	5.94	6.23	6.51	6.77	7.03	7.28	7.51	7.75	7.97	8.19	8.40
9.00	2.58	3.16	3.65	4.08	4.47	4.83	5.16	5.48	5.77	6.06	6.32	6.58	6.83	7.07	7.30	7.53	7.75	7.96	8.16
9.50	2.51	3.08	3.55	3.97	4.35	4.70	5.03	5.33	5.62	5.89	6.16	6.41	6.65	6.88	7.11	7.33	7.54	7.75	7.95
10.00	2.45	3.00	3.46	3.87	4.24	4.58	4.90	5.20	5.48	5.74	6.00	6.24	6.48	6.71	6.93	7.14	7.35	7.55	7.75
10.50	2.39	2.93	3.38	3.78	4.14	4.47	4.78	5.07	5.35	5.61	5.86	6.09	6.32	6.55	6.76	6.97	7.17	7.37	7.56
11.00	2.34	2.86	3.30	3.69	4.05	4.37	4.67	4.95	5.22	5.48	5.72	5.95	6.18	6.40	6.61	6.81	7.01	7.20	7.39
11.50	2.28	2.80	3.23	3.61	3.96	4.27	4.57	4.85	5.11	5.36	5.60	5.82	6.04	6.26	6.46	6.66	6.85	7.04	7.22
12.00	2.24	2.74	3.16	3.54	3.87	4.18	4.47	4.74	5.00	5.24	5.48	5.70	5.92	6.12	6.32	6.52	6.71	6.89	7.07
12.50	2.19	2.68	3.10	3.46	3.79	4.10	4.38	4.65	4.90	5.14	5.37	5.59	5.80	6.00	6.20	6.39	6.57	6.75	6.93
13.00	2.15	2.63	3.04	3.40	3.72	4.02	4.30	4.56	4.80	5.04	5.26	5.48	5.68	5.88	6.08	6.26	6.45	6.62	6.79
13.50	2.11	2.58	2.98	3.33	3.65	3.94	4.22	4.47	4.71	4.94	5.16	5.37	5.58	5.77	5.96	6.15	6.32	6.50	6.67
14.00	2.07	2.54	2.93	3.27	3.59	3.87	4.14	4.39	4.63	4.86	5.07	5.28	5.48	5.67	5.86	6.04	6.21	6.38	6.55
14.50	2.03	2.49	2.88	3.22	3.52	3.81	4.07	4.32	4.55	4.77	4.98	5.19	5.38	5.57	5.75	5.93	6.10	6.27	6.43
15.00	2.00	2.45	2.83	3.16	3.46	3.74	4.00	4.24	4.47	4.69	4.90	5.10	5.29	5.48	5.66	5.83	6.00	6.16	6.32

Formula oz=SQRT((3*(Pachvmetrv-410))/D)

Figure 7-8c. Using the Munnerlyn formula, an optical zone calculation was created. The optical zone chart will give the maximum optical zone possible given a particular corneal thickness and diopter ablation, which will leave a 250 μ depth. The optical zone becomes somewhat limiting in the higher corrections, particularly in corneas of a thickness in the low 500s. (Reprinted with permission from Gimbel HV, Anderson Penno EE. *LASIK Complications: Prevention and Management.* Thorofare, NJ: SLACK Incorporated, 1999.)

REFERENCES

1. Campos M, Carvalho MJ, Scarpi M, Chamon W. Excimer laser intrastromal keratomileusis (LASIK): A clinical follow-up. *Ophthalmic Surgery and Lasers.* 1996(suppl);27(5):S534.

2. Maloney RK. Epithelial ingrowth after lamellar refractive surgery. *Ophthalmic Surgery and Lasers.* 1996(suppl);27(5):S535.

3. Gimbel HV, Levy SG. Indications, results, and complications of LASIK. *Current Opinion in Ophthalmology.* 1998;9;IV;3-8.

4. Stulting RD, Carr JD, Thompson KP, Waring GO, Wiley WM, Walker JG. Complications of laser in situ keratomileusis for the correction of myopia. *Ophthalmology.* 1999;106:13-20.

5. Gimbel HV, Anderson Penno EE, Van Westenbrugge JA, Ferensowicz M, Furlong MT. Incidence and management of intraoperative and early postoperative complications in 1000 consecutive LASIK cases. *Ophthalmology.* 1998;105:1839-1848.

6. Wilson SE. LASIK complications. *Cornea.* 1998;17(5):459-467.

7. Iskander NG, Peters NT, Anderson Penno EE, Gimbel, HV. Postoperative complications in LASIK. *Current Opinion in Ophthalmology.* 2000;11(4):273-279.

8. Çŝker S, Er H, Kahvecioglu C. Laser in situ keratomileusis to correct hyperopia from +4.25 to +8.00 diopters. *J Refract Surg.* 1998;14(1):26-30.

9. Castillo A, Diaz-Valle D, Gutierrez AR, Toledano N, Romero F. Peripheral melt of flap after laser in situ keratomileusis. *J Refract Surg.* 1998;14:61-63.

10. Helena MC, Meisler D, Wilson SE. Epithelial growth within the lamellar interface after laser in situ keratomileusis (LASIK). *Cornea.* 1997;16(3):300-305.

11. Perez-Santonja JJ, Bellot J, Claramonte P, Ismail MM, Alio JL. Laser in situ keratomileusis for correction of high myopia. *J Cataract Refract Surg.* 1997;23:372-385.

12. Cubbitt CL, Lausch RN, Oakes JE. Difference in interleukin 6 gene expression between cultured human corneal epithelial cells and keratocytes. *Invest Ophthalmol Vis Sci.* 1995;36(2):330-336.

13. Goosey J, Samaha A, Vasquez A, Belloso M, Kimbrough M. LASIK for the correction of low, moderate and high myopia. *American Society Cataract and Refractive Surgery. Symposium on Cataract, IOL and Refractive Surgery.* (Abstract #62). 1998.

14. Salah T. Reoperation following LASIK. In: Pallikaris IG, Siganos D, eds. *LASIK.* Thorofare, NJ: SLACK Incorporated; 1998:307.

15. Spivack LD. Results of LASIK using a new nomogram. In: *American Society of Cataract and Refractive Surgery. Symposium on Cataract, IOL, and Refractive Surgery.* (Abstract #10). 1998:37.

16. Suarez E, Cardenas JJ. Intraoperative complications of LASIK. In Buratto L, Brint S, eds. *LASIK: Principles and Techniques.* Thorofare, NJ: SLACK Incorporated: 1998:377.

17. Slade SG. Abnormal induced topography: Central islands. In: Machat JJ, ed. *Excimer Laser Refractive Surgery: Practice and Principles.* Thorofare, NJ: SLACK Incorporated; 1996:399.

18. Waring GO, Thompson KP, Stulting RD, Carr JD. Laser in situ keratomileusis for the correction of myopia in 995 consecutive eyes. *Invest Ophthalmol Vis Sci.* (ARVO Abstract 1084). 1997;38;S231.

19. Probst LE, Machat JJ. LASIK enhancement techniques and results. In: Buratto L, Brint SF, eds. *LASIK: Principles and Techniques.* Thorofare, NJ: SLACK Incorporated; 1998;325-338.

20. Van Westenbrugge JA, Gimbel HV, Kaye GB. Photorefractive keratectomy retreatment. In: Serdarevic ON, ed. *Refractive Surgery: Current Techniques and Management.* New York, NY: Igaku-Shoin; 1997:95-129.

21. Seiler T, Koufala K, Richter G. Iatrogenic keratoconus after laser in situ keratomileusis. *J Refract Surg.* 1998;14:312-317.

22. Geggel HS, Talley AR. Delayed onset keratectasia following laser in situ keratomileusis. *J Cataract Refract Surg.* 1999;25:582-586.

23. Leung ATS, Rao SK, Lam DSC. Delayed onset keratectasia following laser in situ keratomileusis. Letter to the editor. *J Cataract Refract Surg.* 1999;25:1036-1037.

24. Seiler T, Quurke AW. Iatrogenic keratectasia after LASIK in a case of forme fruste keratoconus. *J Cataract Refract Surg.* 1998;24:1007-1009.

25. Wang Z, Chen J, Yang B. Posterior corneal surface topographic changes after laser in situ keratomileusis are related to residual corneal bed thickness. *Ophthalmology.* 1999;106:406-409.

26. Speicher L, Gottinger W. Progressive corneal ectasia after laser in situ keratomileusis. *Klinische Monatsblatter fur Augenheilkunde.* 1998;213:247-251.

27. Reinstein DZ, Srivannaboon S, Sutton HFS, Silverman RH, Holland SP, Coleman DJ. Risk of ectasia in LASIK: Revised safety criteria. *Invest Ophthalmol Vis Sci.* (ARVO Abstract #2121). 1999;40(4):S403.

28. Rao SK, Padmanabhan P. Posterior keratoconus: An expanded classification scheme based on corneal topography. *Ophthalmology.* 1998;105:1206-1212.

8

LASIK Enhancement and Retreatment Concerns

As in all types of refractive surgery, additional surgery may be necessary following LASIK. Reoperations may be needed for treatment of unsatisfactory refractive outcomes (enhancement) or for treatment of complications or quality of vision improvement (retreatment). Enhancements and retreatments may be simple—using the same modality for the primary and secondary surgery, or mixed—using an alternate technique for the secondary surgery (Table 8-1). The majority of enhancements following primary LASIK are likely to be simple enhancements. However, there may be special cases in which a mixed enhancement or retreatment will involve LASIK as the primary or secondary treatment. These are discussed in more detail below.

In combined sequential refractive surgery, a planned approach may include the use of multiple techniques, such as creating a LASIK flap followed by implantation of a phakic IOL such that the flap is available in advance should enhancement be desired.

SIMPLE ENHANCEMENTS

The timing for enhancements in cases of undercorrection, overcorrection, and regression is discussed in Chapter 7. Possible causes and prevention were also pre-

Table 8-1
Enhancement and Retreatment After Previous Refractive Surgery

Simple	Mixed
Simple enhancement (eg, LASIK enhancement following primary LASIK)	Mixed enhancement (eg, LASIK for hyperopia after primary RK)
Simple retreatment (eg, recutting a after primary LASIK)	Mixed retreatment (eg, PTK for flap irregular astigmatism after primary LASIK)

viously discussed in Chapter 7. Regardless of the reason, the surgical techniques involved in lifting the flap for simple enhancement are straightforward. The flap margin should be marked carefully at the slit lamp using a marking pen or the tip of a small instrument, such as a 20-gauge needle (Figures 8-1a and b). A Sinsky hook is used to break adhesions at the flap edge and a forceps is then used to gently peel the flap away from the stromal bed. The same care should be used in handling the flap as is required in primary procedures. The location of the hinge should be confirmed prior to attempted dissection (eg, nasally for the ACS versus superiorly with the Hansatome).

In most cases, the flaps can be lifted in this manner for up to 24 months and longer, as discussed in Chapter 7; however, in some circumstances the flap may be too adherent to dissect and may require that a new flap be cut (see Patient Example 28).

The same principles regarding fluid management discussed in earlier sections apply during enhancements to avoid flap edema or flap shrinkage. When a hyperopic enhancement is performed, the edge of the stromal bed and hinge should be shielded with a sponge, as discussed in Chapter 5, to avoid risk of epithelial ingrowth.

Prior to replacing the flap, epithelial tags and folds should be carefully swept away from the edge of the stromal bed. Meticulous attention to removal of any epithelium or debris from the gutter is essential to avoid epithelial ingrowth. Reapproximating the edges of the epithelium, whether on the flap or outside the flap, must be meticulously performed after flap replacement.

Replacement of the flap, striae test, and careful removal of the drape and speculum should proceed as described for primary LASIK. Because the epithelium at the edges may be slightly more irregular following enhancements (due to dissection and tearing rather than cutting), it is not uncommon for patients to complain of some increased discomfort as compared to their primary surgery. Patients should be reassured that this is to be expected; however, prolonged discomfort or severe pain warrants a slit lamp exam. A detailed outline of primary LASIK technique as performed at our center will follow in Chapter 9. The techniques of laser ablation, flap replacement, and postoperative care apply to enhancements as well as primary LASIK procedures.

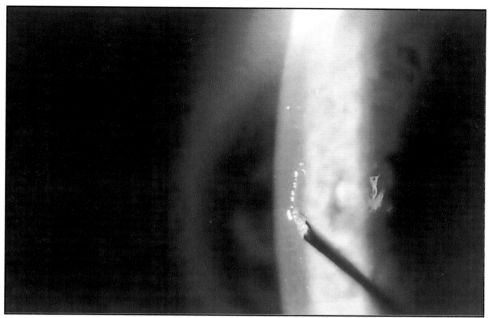

Figure 8-1a. Marking the flap for enhancement. This photograph demonstrates our method for using a 20-gauge needle to mark the edge of the flap at the slit lamp. (Reprinted with permission from Gimbel HV, Anderson Penno EE. *LASIK Complications: Prevention and Management.* Thorofare, NJ: SLACK Incorporated, 1999.)

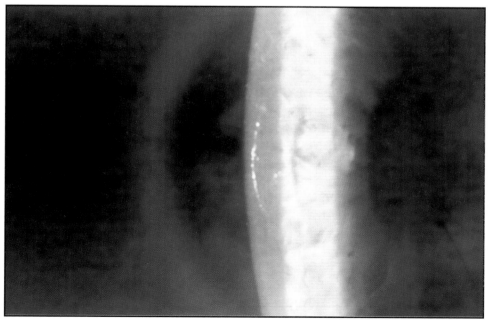

Figure 8-1b. This mark of the edge of the flap margin can be easily located intraoperatively. (Reprinted with permission from Gimbel HV, Anderson Penno EE. *LASIK Complications: Prevention and Management.* Thorofare, NJ: SLACK Incorporated, 1999.)

SIMPLE RETREATMENTS

There are some circumstances in which a recut following primary LASIK is necessary (see Patient Examples 28 and 40). For example, a recut after a buttonhole or partial flap can be done after 3 months. When recutting with a different microkeratome, consideration must be given to using the same depth plate to avoid resulting slivers of tissue (see Patient Example 40). In several cases, we have used the same depth plate for a recut using the Hansatome with good results.

MIXED ENHANCEMENTS

LASIK After Radial Keratotomy

Because of the success of LASIK for myopia astigmatism and hyperopia correction, surgeons around the world are evaluating the use of LASIK for correction of refractive errors particularly hyperopia following myopic radial keratotomy (RK). LASIK does not allow for smoothing of the surface but does reduce the risks associated with a 9 to 9.5 mm debridement of epithelium necessary in photorefractive keratectomy (PRK) (Tables 8-2a and b). There have been reports that haze may occur with a higher incidence if PRK is performed over RK, than when PRK is performed in a primary case (Figure 8-2).[1-2] In addition to haze, slow re-epithelialization, infection, infiltrates, and the uncertain refractive effects of laser ablations of the epithelium if PTK smoothing of the incision ridges is used along with PRK are concerns when treating these eyes with PRK. With careful handling of the flap, the incisions hold together except at times in the periphery of the flap. However, early results are quite promising. The challenge of hyperopic LASIK, whether for primary cases or for hyperopia consecutive to RK, is to obtain a large enough flap with a small enough hinge to allow for the full 9 to 9.5 mm blending treatment zones required for stable hyperopia correction.

A number of LASIK treatments have been performed over previous RK in our center. Concern has been expressed that the flap integrity may be compromised by the radial incisions in these eyes; however, in our experience and that of others, careful handling of the flap has avoided any serious degree of this complication.[3-4] There may be an increased risk of dehiscence of old RK incisions with dissection of the LASIK flap in subsequent enhancement procedures. For this reason, if subsequent enhancements are necessary, a new keratectomy (rather than lifting the old flap) should be considered.

Results of LASIK following RK have been good, although refractive instability and hyperopic shifts due to the RK incisions may persist (see Patient Example 29). In addition, these eyes may show variability in response to the laser. In our experience with hyperopic LASIK after RK, some peripheral incision separation induced astigmatism and flap management problems, but there was no loss of BCVA, and no postoperative haze was noted (Figure 8-3). Epithelial ingrowth in the incisions that separate is also a potential problem.

More research on corneal procedures to reverse RK overcorrection should be carried out. There is currently no surgical method with minimal complications that

Tables 8-2a and b

Correction of Myopia and Hyperopia Following RK

(a)
PRK Advantages vs. LASIK Advantages

PRK	LASIK
•PTK smoothing possible	•Quick recovery
•No incision separation	•Less regression
•No flap adherence complication	•Higher correction possible
•No epithelial ingrowth	

(b)
PRK Disadvantages vs. LASIK Disadvantages

PRK	LASIK
•Haze	•Incision separation
•Regression	•Surface irregularities not corrected
•Less predictable	•Flap instability postop
•Large epithelial debridement	•Retreatment may require recut rather
•Delayed re-epithelialization time	than relifting

(Reprinted with permission from Gimbel HV, Anderson Penno EE. LASIK Complications: Prevention and Management. Thorofare, NJ: SLACK Incorporated, 1999.)

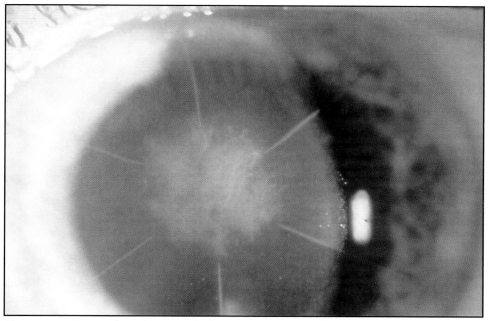

Figure 8-2. Haze. This photograph demonstrates severe haze following myopic PRK over RK. (Reprinted with permission from Gimbel HV, Anderson Penno EE. *LASIK Complications: Prevention and Management.* Thorofare, NJ: SLACK Incorporated, 1999.)

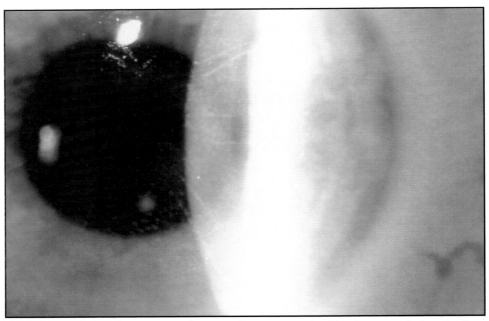

Figure 8-3. Shifted flap (LASIK after RK). One can see in this photograph that the flap incisions are misaligned with the incisions in the bed, indicating that the flap has shifted. When performing LASIK after RK, the alignment of the incisions is a sensitive marker for proper flap position (see Patient Example 26). (Reprinted with permission from Gimbel HV, Anderson Penno EE. *LASIK Complications: Prevention and Management.* Thorofare, NJ: SLACK Incorporated, 1999.)

can be recommended with great confidence for overcorrected RK patients who have not yet developed cataracts. The qualitative differences in the visual and refractive outcomes and the long-term stability of the refraction need to be compared between LASIK and PRK for refractive corrections after RK. Both PRK and LASIK represent useful modalities for the treatment of refractive errors following RK.

LASIK After Epikeratophakia

We have performed two cases of LASIK over epikeratophakia. These were over the nonfreeze Barraquer-Krumeich-Swinger (BKS) epikeratophakia, which was a 9-mm donor button (lenticule) tucked into the dissection beginning at the 6-mm trephination. There was no breakdown of the integrity of the flap by cutting through the different lamellae of the graft and the host. One case resulted in an unexpected overcorrection, suggesting that a conservative approach is warranted, as these eyes may respond unexpectedly to laser ablation. In a subsequent case, the cut was made on the graft, and the flap was put down without laser correction to assess the refractive effect of the cut alone. There was much reduced astigmatism without any laser ablation (see Patient Examples 30 and 31). Our experience is very limited with regard to LASIK after epikeratophakia, but our results have been satisfactory. The risk of haze may also be less with LASIK than with PRK (Figure 8-4).

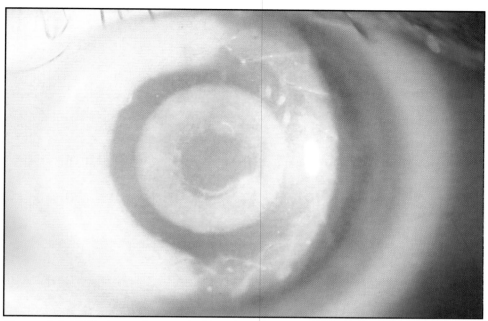

Figure 8-4. PRK after epikeratophakia. This photograph demonstrates haze that was encountered when PRK was performed over epikeratophakia. (Reprinted with permission from Gimbel HV, Anderson Penno EE. *LASIK Complications: Prevention and Management.* Thorofare, NJ: SLACK Incorporated, 1999.)

LASIK After Penetrating Keratoplasty

LASIK has been performed following penetrating keratoplasty (PKP) at our center and by others with good results.[5] Prior to considering a LASIK enhancement, the graft must be well-healed, all sutures removed, and the refraction must be stable (see Patient Example 32). We have had only a few case experiences and learned that a steep cornea is at risk for buttonhole (180 μ depth plate should be used if the cornea is steep or has very high astigmatism).

LASIK After PRK

As a general rule, most surgeons prefer to perform PRK enhancements over PRK. In selected cases, however, LASIK may be considered if the PRK was not for a high correction (in which case the cornea may be too thin for LASIK). Patients at risk for additional haze based on the response to primary PRK may also be treated with LASIK for enhancements (see Patient Example 33). In a recent case at our center, a patient with regression and haze following PRK elected to have LASIK enhancement performed because of a steroid-induced increase in IOP. It was felt that additional PRK treatment without the use of steroids would carry a risk for development of additional haze; therefore, LASIK was performed with good results. In another case of LASIK following myopic PRK, a large central epithelial abrasion occurred from the pass of the microkeratome.

PRK After LASIK

PRK after LASIK is generally not recommended, as lifting the flap for enhancement is quite straightforward. For surface irregularities from wrinkles or flap complications, PTK and PRK may be done if the flap is thin or has been buttonholed. There is, however, an increased risk of haze using PRK (see Patient Example 34). Based on our experience in this one case, we would advise recutting a deeper flap for refractive correction following thin or buttonholed flaps. PTK may be safely used to smooth irregularities on the surface. PRK is, however, an option for patients who have had previous failed attempts at LASIK resulting from a loss of suction or a partial cut.

LASIK After IOL Implantation

LASIK has been used to correct residual refractive error after cataract extraction with IOL implantation at our center, as well as at other centers.[6] In our experience, this has been a safe and effective enhancement procedure following cataract extraction (see Patient Example 35).

SPECIAL CASES

LASIK in Nystagmus

We have performed LASIK in the presence of nystagmus. It is certainly possible to hold the eye very stable with a Thornton ring or a Fine-Thornton ring, stabilizing the head with one hand and then the eye with the other hand, with firm pressure into the head cushion of the chair for stability. It is important not to rotate the eye with the pressure of the Thornton ring, in which case the pupil could still be centered—as the laser beam could still be centered on the pupil but not on the apex of the cornea because of the rotation of the eye. To avoid this, the Thornton ring has to be placed perpendicular to the floor; and when pressure is applied and released as a check of rotation, one can determine whether the ring is being applied perpendicularly. With this technique, rotation is avoided because there should be no movement of the eye upon release of the ring during this testing maneuver if the Thornton ring is placed properly. In addition, if a high correction is being performed, it is well to pause and reconfirm that there is no rotation of the eye on one or more occasions through the laser application. This maneuver is also used when patients cannot maintain a stable fixation because of micro and macro saccades that are uncontrollable on the part of the patient (see Patient Example 41).

Unilateral Surgery/Anisometropia

For the most part, it may be advisable to match the procedures in the two eyes (ie, LASIK bilaterally, PRK bilaterally, or refractive lensectomy bilaterally) as there may be differences in the qualities of the vision with different refractive procedures. However, there may be some cases in which the procedure in the fellow eye is not matched. In rare cases, it may be necessary to modify or change the approach in the fellow eye, for example if a complication is encountered during or following surgery on the first eye, as was encountered in Patient Example 36.

There has been debate in the literature as to the advisability of performing bilateral same-day surgery; however, our experience, as well as that of others, has indicated that bilateral surgery is indeed safe and is in many ways preferable to unilateral surgery.[7-8] In the occasional case in which the patient requests to have one eye done at a time, there have been significant complaints of visual discomfort relating to anisometropia if a contact lens cannot be worn in the fellow eye. This has also occurred in circumstances where the first eye in a bilateral case was performed without complications, and a complication occurred in the second eye that resulted in no laser ablation in the fellow eye. These patients also complain of significant anisometropia that is severe enough that it may be difficult to perform their daily tasks. In cases where there is a flap complication in the second eye with resulting anisometropia (ie, a buttonhole in the second eye that results in an inability to perform the laser ablation), we advise waiting as long as possible before considering a contact lens correction in the eye that had the complication. We have started patients on a contact lens as early as 1 week following a buttonhole with careful instructions with regard to placing and/or removing the contact lens. The patients have been instructed to use liberal wetting drops and to come to the clinic for removal of the contact lens should they encounter any problems whatsoever when attempting to remove the contact lens. With careful education and detailed instructions, we have had no complications relating to the use of contact lenses following flap complications; however, a conservative approach is warranted, and if the patient is able to function satisfactorily without contact lens correction of the fellow eye, we advise waiting as long as possible.

CONCLUSION

Refractive surgeons must be familiar with techniques of simple enhancements as well as mixed enhancements and retreatments. Further discussion of this topic can be found in Chapter 15 of *Refractive Surgery: A Manual of Principles and Practice*.

REFERENCES

1. Suarez E, Cardenas JJ. Intraoperative complications of LASIK. In: Buratto L, Brint S, eds. *LASIK: Principles and Techniques*. Thorofare, NJ: SLACK Incorporated; 1998:377.

2. Seiler T, Jean B. Photorefractive keratectomy to correct residual myopia after radial keratotomy. *J Refract Corneal Surg*. 1992;8:211-214.

3. Gutierrez AM. Reoperations with the excimer laser. In: Buratto L, Brint S, eds. *LASIK: Principles and Techniques*. Thorofare, NJ: SLACK Incorporated; 1998:344.

4. Thompson V. Flap management during LASIK after radial keratotomy. Letter. *J Refract Surg*. 1997;13:128.

5. Ditzen K, Huschka H, Pieger S. Laser in situ keratomileusis for hyperopia. *J Cataract Refract Surg*. 1998;24(1):42-47.

6. Stulting RD, Carr JD, Thompson HP, Wiley W, Waring III GO. Laser in-situ keratomileusis for the correction of myopia after previous ocular surgery. In: American Society of Cataract and Refractive Surgery. *Symposium on Cataract, IOL, and Refractive Surgery*. (Abstract #144). 1998:37.

7. Hardten DR, Chu YR, Preschel N, Jedlicka J, Lindstrom RL. Bilateral LASIK: Results and safety in a randomized prospective study. In: American Society of Cataract and Refractive Surgery. *Symposium on Cataract, IOL, and Refractive Surgery.* (Abstract #134). 1998:34.

8. Vicary D, Page G, Sun X. Bilateral simultaneous LASIK in 228 eyes. In: American Society of Cataract and Refractive Surgery. *Symposium on Cataract, IOL, and Refractive Surgery.* (Abstract #135). 1998:34.

9

LASIK Techniques

The fundamental principles of complication-free LASIK surgery are adequate exposure, attention to details, timing, fluid management (minimize drying, minimize hydration), feather-touch gentleness, and careful inspection of the flap, the epithelium, and the interface.

Our technique has been developed using the ACS and further refined using the Hansatome and the Nidek EC-5000 laser system. It is imperative to be familiar with the particular features of the microkeratome and laser system being used, because there may be nuances that may vary from system to system. The following is a step-by-step outline of the LASIK procedure as it is done at our center.

FINAL PREOPERATIVE DISCUSSION AND INFORMED CONSENT

Preoperative testing, patient education, informed consent, and patient selection are discussed at length in Chapter 2. Detailed discussions including corneal topography, advanced examination techniques, and comanagement of refractive surgery patients can be found in Chapters 4, 5, and 6 in *Refractive Surgery: A Manual of Principles and Practice.*

Just prior to surgery, the surgeon must carefully review the patient's records. The surgeon should review with the patient the risks, benefits, alternatives, and

Figure 9-1. Patient identification sticker. (Reprinted with permission from Gimbel HV, Anderson Penno EE. *LASIK Complications: Prevention and Management.* Thorofare, NJ: SLACK Incorporated, 1999.)

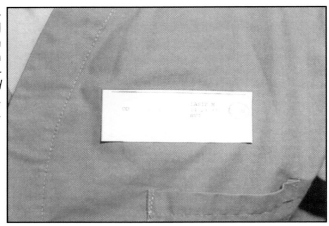

Figure 9-2. Surgeon reference card. This card, with salient patient information, is placed above the microscope for use as a quick reference for the surgeon. (Reprinted with permission from Gimbel HV, Anderson Penno EE. *LASIK Complications: Prevention and Management.* Thorofare, NJ: SLACK Incorporated, 1999.)

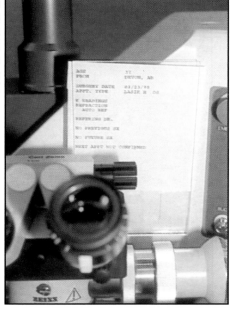

expectations of surgery. After the discussion with the patient, the informed consent should be signed. Each patient is given an identification sticker noting the eye and the planned procedure (Figure 9-1). This information is also entered on a card above the microscope of the laser as a quick reference for the surgeon (Figure 9-2). The laser parameters are then calculated and double-checked (Figure 9-3). It is a important to double-check the astigmatic axis laser parameter against the topography. The parameters are then entered into the laser and double-checked by a second nurse or technician and the surgeon. Patient sedation is minimized to avoid problems with fixation. Preoperative anesthetic drops are also minimized to avoid softening of epithelium, which may lead to epithelial complications.

Gimbel Eye Centre LASIK Worksheet

Patient Name: _____ _____ Age: _____

Surgery Date: _____ Eye: _____ Dom: _____ Sx: 1st 2nd bilat

If enh, over which procedure: PRK   LASIK   RK   AK   lensectomy   Enhancement #: _____

If enh, reason: overresponse underresponse progression   regression haze C.I.   mono-vision reversal

1. Pre-op Manifest Refraction: _____ - _____ x _____   Previous laser used: _____

2. Pre-op Cyclo Refraction: _____ - _____ x _____

3. Desired Refractive Change: _____ - _____ x _____   Average K's: _____ V.D.: _____

4. Targeted Refraction: _____ - _____ x _____   Corneal Diam.: _____ Monovision? Y N

5. Desired Ref. Change Plus Cyl: _____ + _____ x _____   Pupil Size: light _____ dim _____

Cylinder	**Myopia**	**Hyperopia**
Refractive cyl _____	Sphere: - _____	Calibration Factor: _____
x _____ % → subtract cyl. effect: _____		Sphere: + _____
Laser parameter cyl _____	Adjusted sphere: - _____ →	add plus cyl. effect: _____
x _____ %	att/ach factor _____ %	Adjusted sphere: + _____
Cylinder effect on sphere _____ → Laser parameter sphere: - _____		att/ach factor _____ %
		Laser parameter sphere: + _____

Laser Parameter A: _____ - _____ x _____   Tx Zone: _____ mm Tran Zone: _____ mm

B: _____ - _____ x _____   Tx Zone: _____ mm Tran Zone: _____ mm

C: _____ - _____ x _____   Tx Zone: _____ mm Tran Zone: _____ mm

Axis: □ Corneal map   □ Manual K's   □ Manifest refraction   □ Cyclo refraction

Surgeon initial: _____   Laser used: Nidek _____ Serial # _____, Other _____

CMS Computer Data Entry: _____ - _____ x _____ (Total of all zones)   Tech. initial: _____

Data Entry Verified by: _____ Microkeratome Data: □ Chiron, □ Other _____ Serial Number: _____

Lateral canthotomy?   Yes   No   Extra Irrigation?   Yes   No   Edge?   Yes   No

Suction Time: _____ Between Time: _____ Laser Time: _____ Total Sx Time: _____

Time Between Replacing Flap and Verifying Adherence with the Striae Test: _____ Stop/Start Time: _____

Flap Diameter: _____ mm Hinge Length: _____ mm Corneal Diameter: _____ mm

Patient Stability: _____ Centration: _____ Epi Adherence: _____ Surface Quality: _____ Gutter Width: _____

(Rate 1-4; 4=good, 1=poor)   CALIBRATION DATA:

Comments: PMMA #: _____

Box # (-3.0) _____

Box # (exp zone) _____

Box # (hyperopic) _____

Hyp cut (sph) _____

Surgeon: _____   Laser Tech Signature: _____

Figure 9-3. This is an example of a calculation worksheet used for LASIK. As software or algorithms are modified, the worksheet is modified. It includes information on suction time, surgery time, and other parameters, which are entered into the computer for each patient so that these parameters can be retrieved at a later date for ongoing studies. (Reprinted with permission from Gimbel HV, Anderson Penno EE. *LASIK Complications: Prevention and Management.* Thorofare, NJ: SLACK Incorporated, 1999.)

INTRAOPERATIVE TECHNIQUES

The suction ring and microkeratome are inspected and run through a series of checks under the microscope by the surgeon or designated nurse assistant. Each microkeratome is checked according to specific criteria (see Chapter 3) (Figures 9-4a, b, c, and 9-5). All parts are checked for tightness. The blade is inspected under the microscope. The gears are then inspected and manually checked for freedom of movement. Blade movement is visually confirmed. The suction ring and suction port are inspected for debris or BSS crystals (see Figure 9-5). Regardless of the microkeratome in use, the microkeratome is seated on the suction ring, and full movement (forward and reverse) is confirmed prior to each case.

The patient is then positioned on the bed perpendicular to the laser, head not turned or tilted, and a pedestal support is placed under the head to minimize movement from pulse pressure. As in all types of ocular surgery, proper head position should be obtained prior to commencing to avoid difficulties with exposure. The patient is draped carefully to avoid creation of a pseudopalpebral fissure (Figure 9-6). The choice of speculum is a locking or strong spring, and the head is positioned slightly chin-up for maximum exposure (lateral canthotomy to be performed as needed). The fellow eye is patched, and a gauze sponge is placed to catch any fluid (Figure 9-7). The patient is instructed as to fixation lights and is instructed not to move arms and legs as this will move the head. Also, instruct the patient to keep the fellow eye open, and to blink normally but not to squeeze. Patients have the option of listening to commentary as the surgery proceeds (Figure 9-8).

Straight gentian violet marks are placed in an asymmetric pattern and/or two different circle marks are used to aid in repositioning and in the event of a free cap. Excess gentian violet is removed gently with a damp sponge. The surgeon locates the foot switch and has the toe ready on the forward button. The suction ring is firmly placed before suction is applied and held firmly until scleral indentation occurs. Attachment is achieved once suction is applied. Initial placement of the suction ring should anticipate the extra shift nasally with the ACS superiorly or with the Hansatome (in some eyes) as the ring seats when suction is applied. The patient should be advised that the vision will dim or go black. Some patients may still see a small amount of light just as the pass is beginning.

Once suction has been applied, the IOP is measured with the Barraquer tonometer. Prior to placing the tonometer on the cornea, the cornea should be quite damp in order to avoid epithelium sticking to the tonometer.

The IOP should be more than 65 mmHg to avoid thin flaps and buttonholes with the 160 μ plate. To ensure maintenance of good pressure, hold the suction ring steady; it should not be bumped or jiggled. The IOP should be remeasured after any manipulations of lid, drape, or speculum. When seating the microkeratome, it may help to avoid downward pressure and rotate the suction ring and globe slightly to clear the lower lid. Some surgeons then place firm downward pressure as the pass is made.

Just prior to placing the microkeratome, advise the patient that there will be noise and vibration as the microkeratome pass is performed. During the micro-

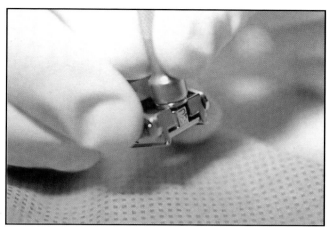

Figure 9-4a. This illustrates proper insertion of the microkeratome depth plate in the ACS head. (Reprinted with permission from Gimbel HV, Anderson Penno EE. *LASIK Complications: Prevention and Management.* Thorofare, NJ: SLACK Incorporated, 1999.)

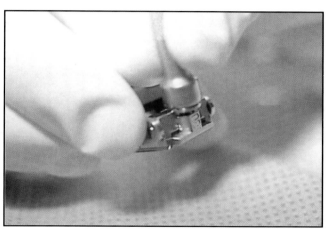

Figure 9-4b. This illustrates incomplete placement of the microkeratome depth plate in the ACS head. (Reprinted with permission from Gimbel HV, Anderson Penno EE. *LASIK Complications: Prevention and Management.* Thorofare, NJ: SLACK Incorporated, 1999.)

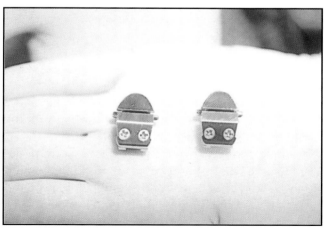

Figure 9-4c. The Chiron Hansatome has the 180 µm and 160-µm depth plates in separate heads. (Reprinted with permission from Gimbel HV, Anderson Penno EE. *LASIK Complications: Prevention and Management.* Thorofare, NJ: SLACK Incorporated, 1999.)

Figure 9-5. Photograph of our standard LASIK equipment setup.

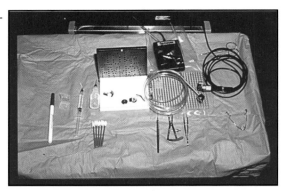

Figure 9-6. To ensure adequate exposure, the standard 3M 1020 ophthalmic drape is cut as demonstrated, and draping techniques are carefully followed (as described in Chapter 5). (Reprinted with permission from Gimbel HV, Anderson Penno EE. *LASIK Complications: Prevention and Management.* Thorofare, NJ: SLACK Incorporated, 1999.)

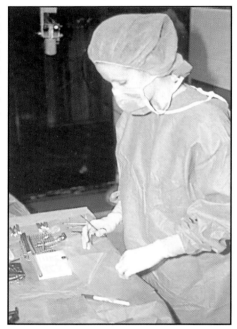

Figure 9-7. The fellow eye is patched, and a gauze sponge is taped to the patient's temple to eliminate any fluid draining from the surgical field, which may cause the patient discomfort.

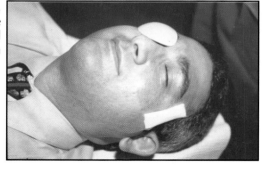

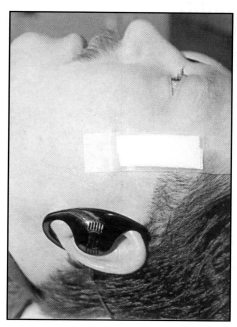

Figure 9-8. To alleviate anxiety, patients may choose to listen to commentary provided through an earpiece as the surgery proceeds. (Reprinted with permission from Gimbel HV, Anderson Penno EE. *LASIK Complications: Prevention and Management.* Thorofare, NJ: SLACK Incorporated, 1999.)

keratome pass, the assistant holds down the speculum to aid in proptosing the globe and avoid interference from the lids or speculum (Figure 9-9). The surgeon should wet the cornea and tracks generously with a moist (nonsaline) sponge prior to engaging the microkeratome to aid in obtaining a smooth cut. Avoid flooding the field with excess irrigation, as excess fluid wicks its way to the motor shaft and deposits salts. The track is checked to make sure that it is clear with no lid, conjunctiva, or drape in the way. The pass should occur forward to the stop without pauses. The microkeratome is then reversed. With the corneal shaper, the surgeon may watch the flap retract out of microkeratome (corneal shaper). The surgeon removes the Hansatome from the suction ring, then turns suction off. For the ACS, the suction is turned off, and the ring and microkeratome assembly are lifted from the eye together.

Centration and focus should be ready before turning the flap. Moisture must not be introduced underneath the flap. The flap is lifted with forceps and placed on a cut sponge or Gimbel-Chayet drape (Figures 9-10a and b). The surgeon must be prepared at this point to make the difficult decision to not proceed if there is any question about flap or bed integrity. Timing is critical to avoid excess drying of flap or bed. At our center, once the flap is lifted, the time between turning the flap and commencing laser ablation is recorded and tabulated for outcomes analysis. No moisture is put on the flap (some surgeons using slower scanning spot lasers do use moisture or viscous agents on the flap). The flap is carefully positioned in a cup position to avoid wrinkles that can imprint on the epithelium and make differentiation from the flap wrinkles difficult.

Positioning of the patient with either hand or foot controls and/or holding the head can be done prior to and during the ablation. Note that dark irides can make

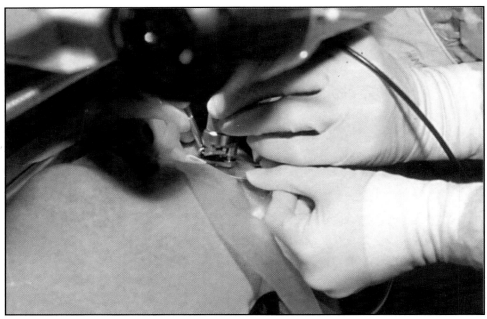

Figure 9-9. During the microkeratome pass, the assistant gently provides downward pressure on the speculum to proptose the globe and aid in exposure. (Reprinted with permission from Gimbel HV, Anderson Penno EE. *LASIK Complications: Prevention and Management.* Thorofare, NJ: SLACK Incorporated, 1999.)

Figure 9-10a. Gimbel-Chayet sponge. The Chayet sponge is modified as demonstrated and placed as discussed in Chapter 5 to absorb bleeding from vessels located in the hinge area and help to avoid blood flowing onto the stromal bed. The tail of the sponge may be used to shield the hinge if necessary. (Reprinted with permission from Gimbel HV, Anderson Penno EE. *LASIK Complications: Prevention and Management.* Thorofare, NJ: SLACK Incorporated, 1999.)

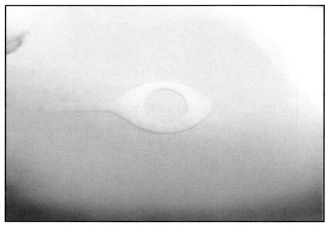

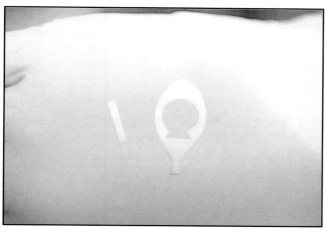

Figure 9-10b. Gimbel-Chayet sponge. The Chayet sponge is modified as demonstrated and placed as discussed in Chapter 5 to absorb bleeding from vessels located in the hinge area and help to avoid blood flowing onto the stromal bed. The tail of the sponge may be used to shield the hinge if necessary. (Reprinted with permission from Gimbel HV, Anderson Penno EE. *LASIK Complications: Prevention and Management.* Thorofare, NJ: SLACK Incorporated, 1999.)

visualization of the pupil difficult; and in this circumstance, the gooseneck side light is helpful. The slit beam on the Nidek may also be helpful in lighting up the iris. The patient is reminded to concentrate on the fixation target, to keep the fellow eye open, and not to swallow or to move arms or legs. It may be helpful to remind the patient that the target may become blurry and the light may seem to move around but to continue looking at the center of the light. The surgeon may need to stabilize the patient's eye with a Thornton ring or modification thereof, using care to avoid rotating the globe with the fixation ring.

After any hyperopic ablation, PTK smoothing is performed to smooth the bed and decrease the likelihood of haze and regression. The bed is moistened with Laservis (Chemedica SA, Vouvry, Switzerland) using a Merocel sponge and the excess fluid is wiped away with a spatula. PTK smoothing for 2 μ is then performed.

To reposition the flap, flip it over onto a dry stromal bed using slight applanating pressure if the epithelium is well attached. Irrigation is used to remove bubbles from under the flap edges (only if bubbles are only at the edge—to avoid hydrating the stroma). The flap should then be hydrated to reform its normal contour and floated into position. Try to avoid debris floating up from the cul-de-sac due to excess irrigation under the flap. A short stroke at the hinge with the cannula parallel to the hinge will remove any folding there and help to position the flap. At this time, observe that the marks are aligned. A Merocel sponge tip soaked in sodium hyaluronate is used to barely touch and caress the flap, starting at the hinge and proceeding in a centripetal manner to remove fluid as soon as possible to avoid hydration of corneal tissues. Remove any interface blood or debris noted at this time, as described in Chapter 5. Do not confuse tiny air bubbles with debris.

Once the flap is in good position, remember to use the variety of inspection techniques available. When using the Nidek EC-5000, the slit lamp can be used for retroillumination as well as direct illumination. The coaxial light can be mixed with the slit beam and used to inspect for surface quality and flap wrinkles. The striae test may be performed after 1.5 to 2.5 minutes. There is variability in the amount of time surgeons wait to ensure adherence of the flap (2 to 4 minutes). Some surgeons do not remove the speculum before 4 minutes in any case. Once adherence of the flap is confirmed, the surgeon can proceed with careful removal of the speculum and drape after drops are placed (Figures 9-11a and b). Steroid, nonsteroidal anti-inflammatory, antibiotic, and viscous drops are placed. The patient is instructed not to squeeze the eyes shut and to look straight ahead. The surgeon holds the lids open while removing the drapes and speculum. The patient is then told to blink normally while the surgeon is inspecting the flap. A bandage contact lens is applied if a large area of epithelium has a been torn or disrupted.

POSTOPERATIVE CARE

Airtight, self-adhesive moisture chambers are placed with instructions not to remove them until at home. Patients are also instructed to reapply them at night or while napping for 1 week. Detailed postoperative instructions include what to expect in terms of burning, light sensitivity, possible foreign body sensation, and foggy vision. An inspection of the flap at the slit lamp 30 minutes after surgery is performed for flaps with horizontal hinges. Flaps are not checked after Hansatome cuts because of the superior hinge. Remember the variety of techniques that can be used at the slit lamp: sclerotic scatter, direct, retroillumination.

CONCLUSION

LASIK is a good technique for the correction of refractive errors and is safe if performed with care on patients who have undergone appropriate preoperative testing and counseling. The principles to keep in mind during all steps of the procedure are attention to detail, consistent timing, and careful fluid management.

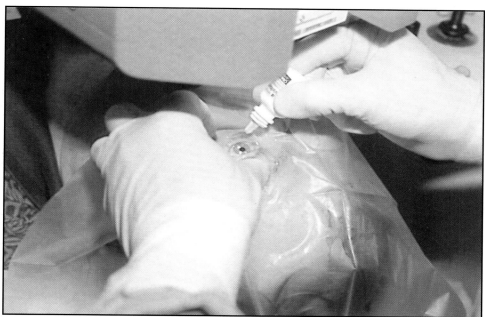

Figure 9-11a. Removal of drapes and speculum. The lids are stabilized with the thumb and forefinger to avoid shifted flaps while drapes and speculum are removed to avoid squeezing of the lids. (Reprinted with permission from Gimbel HV, Anderson Penno EE. *LASIK Complications: Prevention and Management.* Thorofare, NJ: SLACK Incorporated, 1999.)

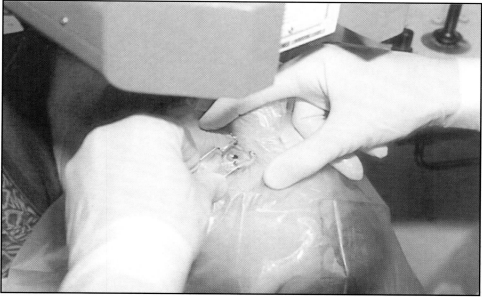

Figure 9-11b. Removal of drapes and speculum. The lids are stabilized with the thumb and forefinger to avoid shifted flaps while drapes and speculum are removed to avoid squeezing of the lids. (Reprinted with permission from Gimbel HV, Anderson Penno EE. *LASIK Complications: Prevention and Management.* Thorofare, NJ: SLACK Incorporated, 1999.)

Section II

Patient Examples

Unless specifically stated otherwise, the microkeratome used in the Patient Examples was a Chiron ACS. Some of these complications may be unique to this microkeratome. Each microkeratome has its own unique benefits and complications. The authors can only describe complications encountered with the system used personally.

Section II Contents

PATIENT EXAMPLE 1

Keratoconus Found on Preoperative Assessment

This 56-year-old woman has a history of discomfort with contacts and frequently changing prescriptions. Her general health was good, and she took no medications. Cycloplegic refraction revealed -0.75 -2.00 x 90 best corrected to 20/25[-2] OD (right eye) and +0.75 -4.75 x 101 best corrected to 20/30[-1] OS (left eye). Manual keratometry revealed 43.00 @ 59 x 44.50 @ 149 OD and 41.25 @ 114 x 45.00 @ 23 OS . It was noted that keratometry mires were distorted. The corneal maps showed inferior steepening consistent with keratoconus. Her IOP was normal. The slit lamp exam revealed 2 to 3 + NS OU (both eyes), and the dilated funduscopic exam was normal.

Due to the presence of keratoconus on corneal mapping, it was felt that a lensectomy with a toric IOL might be an option; however, the patient was informed that her refraction may continue to change, and she elected to continue with contact lenses in the interim. The patient decided that she wanted to wait until her cataracts worsened prior to proceeding with lensectomy. The accompanying corneal maps demonstrate the presence of inferior steepening OU consistent with keratoconus.

To date, keratoconus has been a contraindication to corneal refractive surgery. There is some concern with regard to refractive instability as well as risk of induced corneal ectasia with refractive surgery. Recently, some surgeons have reported that corneal refractive surgery may be an alternative to corneal transplant in patients who are unable to tolerate contact lenses and in whom spectacle correction is suboptimal.[1] The surgeon must review the preoperative data carefully and thoroughly discuss findings, surgical options, and risks of surgery with each patient. Many patients are aware that there may be alternatives to LASIK or PRK, such as phakic IOLs and refractive lensectomy, and regardless of whether or not they proceed with surgery they appreciate being informed of their options.

(Text and figures reprinted with permission from Gimbel HV, Anderson Penno EE. *LASIK Complications: Prevention and Management.* Thorofare, NJ: SLACK Incorporated, 1999.)

---

1. Buzard K. Treatment of mild to moderate keratoconus by LASIK. In: American Society of Cataract and Refractive Surgery. *Symposium on Cataract, IOL, and Refractive Surgery.* (Abstract #73). 1998;19.

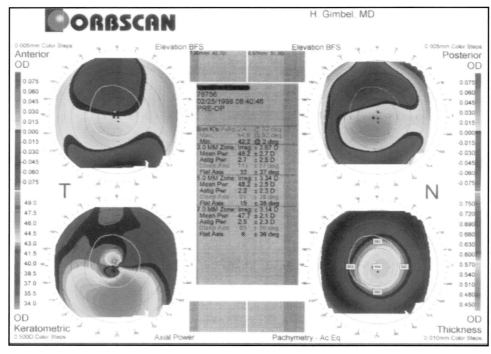

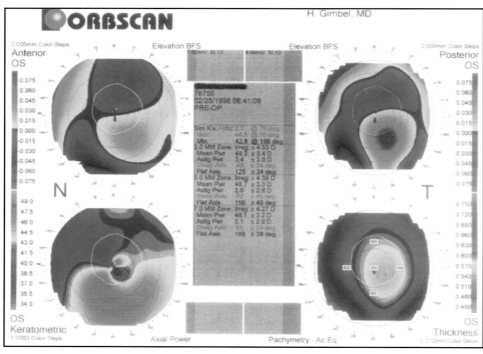

PATIENT EXAMPLE 2

Pellucid Marginal Degeneration Found on Refractive Assessment

This is a 62-year-old man who was left-eye dominant with no previous eye history. His general health was good, and he took no medications. His vision without correction was 20/40⁻¹ OD and 20/300 OS. Manifest refraction was +1.00 -2.50 x 103 best corrected to 20/20 OD and manifest of -2.50 -1.25 x 73 best corrected to 20/15⁻³ OS. Keratometry was 42.87 @ 90, 44.75 @ 4 OD and 45.00 @ 85, 46.25 @ 175 OS. It was noted OD that the axis on keratometry was not perpendicular. Corneal diameters were 11.50 mm OU. The slit lamp exam revealed thinning and inferior bulging of the cornea OD and 1+ posterior subcapsular cataract OS. The corneal map showed classic pellucid patterns OD.

These findings were discussed with the patient. It was explained to the patient that corneal refractive surgery would be a high risk OD due to the pellucid marginal degenerative changes. It was also explained that, because of the presence of the subcapsular cataract, it might be wise to wait and consider lensectomy with an IOL implant at a later date.

This is a case in which the surgeon should advise against corneal refractive surgery. Careful discussion of the underlying pathology (in this case cataracts and pellucid degeneration) and effects on vision and refraction should be included in any discussion of options. Referrals should be made for treatment of any underlying pathology if necessary.

The accompanying corneal maps demonstrate a normal contour OS and the presence of ring cylinder inferiorly OD, which is consistent with pellucid marginal degeneration OS.

(Text and figures [with the exception of the third figure] reprinted with permission from Gimbel HV, Anderson Penno EE. *LASIK Complications: Prevention and Management.* Thorofare, NJ: SLACK Incorporated, 1999.)

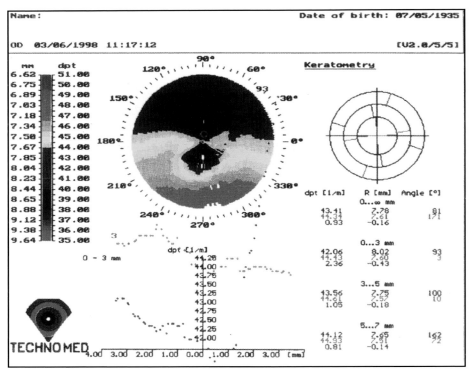

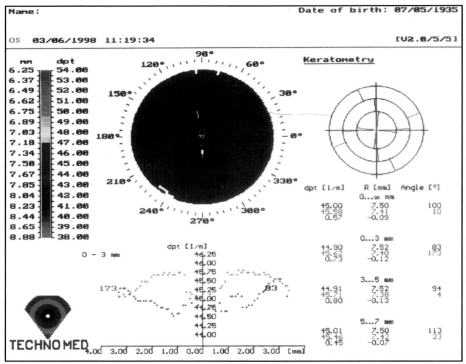

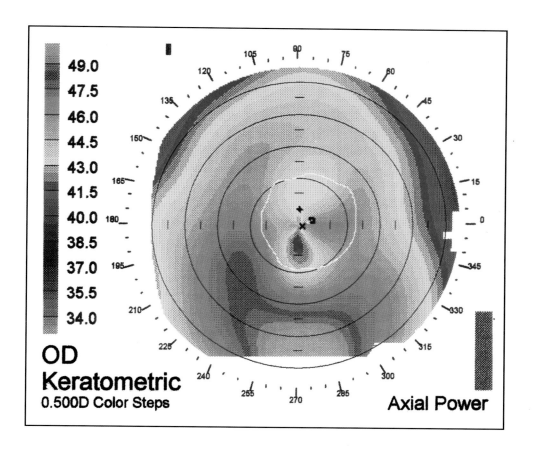

49.0
47.5
46.0
44.5
43.0
41.5
40.0
38.5
37.0
35.5
34.0

OD
Keratometric
0.500D Color Steps

Axial Power

PATIENT EXAMPLE 3

Unmasking of Cylinder

This 43-year-old woman had a history of soft contact lens use, which was discontinued 1 year ago. She has no other medical or ocular problems. Uncorrected vision was count fingers at 2 meters OU. Cycloplegic refraction was 4.25 sphere with vision of 20/20 OD and -4.00 sphere with vision 20/20 OS. Pachymetry was normal, and manual keratometry was 47.00 @ 180 x 47.75 @ 90 OD and 46.75 @ 2 x 47.75 @ 92 OS. The slit lamp and funduscopic exams were within normal. It was noted that there was 0.75 cylinder on manual keratometry and 1.23 D cylinder on the map OD. The left eye was noted to have 1.0 D of cylinder on manual keratometry and 1.23 D on the map. The decision was made to proceed with a spherical correction OU based on the refraction. At 1 month after uncomplicated LASIK surgery, the uncorrected vision was 20/25[-1] OD and 20/20[-1] OS. Manifest refraction was plano -0.50 x 157 OD best corrected to 20/15[-1] and 0.50 -0.75 x 168 OS best corrected to 20/15[-2]. Postoperative keratometry was 42.75 @ 175 x 43.75 @ 85 OD and 42.50 @ 5 x 44.25 @ 95. The patient was very pleased with her vision at this time.

In the accompanying preoperative and postoperative maps, one can see that the degree in axis of corneal cylinder is similar for both eyes preoperatively and postoperatively. In these cases, it can be difficult to decide whether or not to treat cylinder. A conservative approach may be advisable because the patient (as in this case) may be satisfied in spite of a small amount of residual astigmatism; and furthermore, an enhancement can be performed at a later date. Although corneal astigmatism may be present, there may also be a lenticular component. In some cases, the opposite may be true—more cylinder on the refraction than on maps and keratometry. In all cases, a conservative approach is recommended, and the patient may be advised that he or she might be more likely to need an enhancement.

(Text and figures reprinted with permission from Gimbel HV, Anderson Penno EE. *LASIK Complications: Prevention and Management.* Thorofare, NJ: SLACK Incorporated, 1999.)

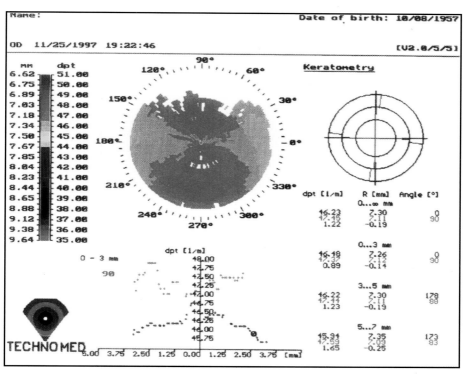

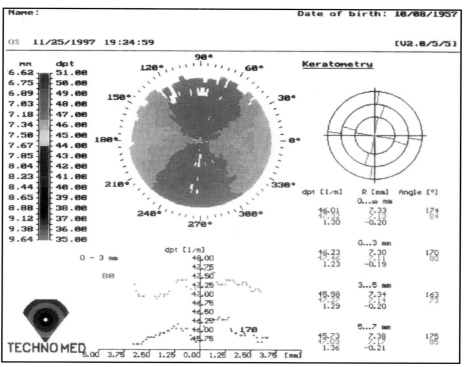

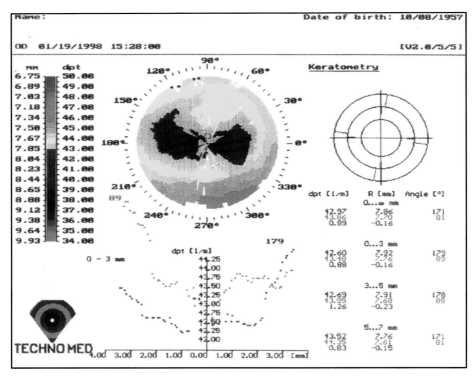

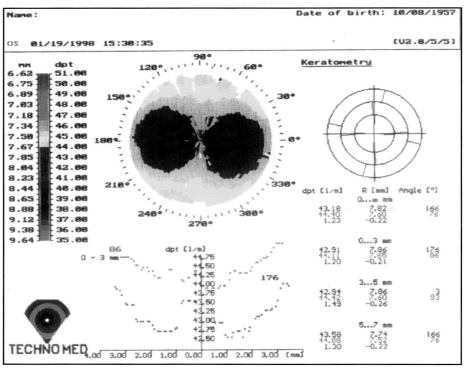

PATIENT EXAMPLE 4

Buttonhole/Inadequate Exposure/Lateral Canthotomy

This 42-year-old woman had a 2-year history of soft contact lens wear. She was on Premarin (Wyeth-Ayerst Laboratories, Philadelphia, Pa), Restoril (Sandoz Pharmaceuticals, East Hanover, NJ), Fiorinal (Sandoz Pharmaceuticals), and had a history of back surgery and a hysterectomy. She had no other medical conditions. Her vision without correction was 20/20⁻² OD and 20/100 OS. Manifest refraction was +1.75 -0.50 x 15 corrected to 20/20⁻² OD and +5.25 -1.25 x 30 corrected to 20/30+2 OS. Cycloplegic refraction was +2.50 -0.50 x 15 best corrected to 20/20-2 OD and +5.50 -1.00 x 30 best corrected to 20/40 OS. Pachymetry was within normal, and manual keratometry revealed 45.75 @ 6 x 47.12 @ 96 OD and 45.75 @ 13 x 47.75 @ 103 OS. The slit lamp and dilated funduscopic exam were within normal. The patient was amblyopic OS.

LASIK OS was performed with the ACS without complications; however, it was necessary to do a lateral canthotomy to make room for the suction ring. At 2 months postoperatively, the patient was happy with her vision OS. Her uncorrected vision was 20/50⁻¹ with a manifest refraction of plano -0.25 @ 65 best corrected to 20/30⁻². It was noted that there was trace scattered haze at the flap interface.

LASIK OD was done with the ACS (also requiring a lateral canthotomy), and a buttonhole was created; therefore, laser ablation was not done. The flap was carefully replaced, and a contact lens was placed.

Three days postoperatively, VASC was 20/70⁻² OD, and the patient complained of multiple images. Manifest refraction was of no help. Eleven days postoperatively, her vision VASC OD was 20/100, manifest refraction showed +2.50 -0.50 x 72 best corrected to 20/60⁻¹. At the slit lamp, it was felt that the central cornea was somewhat distorted and that flap repositioning should be performed. The patient was taken to the operating room, and gentian violet marker was used to make three marks on the temporal side of the flap. A 4-mm zone marker coated with gentian violet was then used to mark the superior and nasal edge of the flap. The flap was lifted with a colibri, and epithelial strands at the flap edges, as well as the buttonhole edges, were removed using a Paton spatula (Bausch & Lomb Surgical, Claremont, Calif). The flap was irrigated using a 30-gauge cannula and smoothed down with a sodium hyaluronate-coated sponge. The edge of the buttonhole was smoothed out with a Paton spatula. After waiting 7 minutes 43 seconds, the striae test using a colibri verified adherence. Drops were placed, and a bandage contact lens was applied. A moisture chamber was then placed over the eye, and the patient left the operating room in good condition.

At 2 weeks postoperatively from the repositioning, VASC OD was 20/50⁻², and the patient complained of multiple images. The manifest refraction was of no help. The cornea revealed 1+ epithelial edema, and a faint edge of the buttonhole was visible superiorly. There was 1+ superficial punctate keratopathy.

Eight months after flap repositioning, UCVA was 20/40, and the manifest refraction revealed +1.75 -0.75 x 50 with a manifest vision of 20/20⁻¹.

The corneal maps demonstrate the appearance of this patient's right eye preoperatively, 1 week postoperatively, 6 days after repositioning, and 5 months postrepositioning. This patient's eyes are pictured in Figures 5-6 and 6-4. Ten months postoperatively, the refraction had stabilized at +2.50 -0.50 x 174 corrected to 20/25[-1]. A new flap was recut using a Hansatome microkeratome and 180 µ depth plate uneventfully. Postoperative day 1 the UCVA was 20/40 with no improvement on manifest refraction. Corneal topography was performed (Map #5). The patient's UCVA gradually improved and by 1 year after recutting, the UCVA was 20/25[+1] with a manifest refraction of +0.50 -0.50 x 161 corrected to 20/20[-1]. Corneal topography is included.

This case illustrates in the first eye (OS) that inadequate exposure may require a lateral canthotomy and that this may allow the case to proceed without complication. Lateral canthotomy may, however, be a risk factor for flap shift, as occurred in this patient's right eye at 3 days postoperatively. The average keratometry readings in this case were 46.44 D OD and 46.75 D OS, which we have learned is a risk factor for buttonholes. We have proceeded without complication in corneas as steep as 52.00 D, indicating that there are additional factors that must come into play (possibly corneal elasticity, corneal diameter, and type of microkeratome in use). Thus, steep corneas are not a contraindication to LASIK, but these patients should be warned of the increased risk and the surgeon should consider using a deeper depth plate. Furthermore, with proper management, BCVA can be preserved.

(Text and figures [with the exception of the fifth and sixth figures] reprinted with permission from Gimbel HV, Anderson Penno EE. *LASIK Complications: Prevention and Management.* Thorofare, NJ: SLACK Incorporated, 1999.)

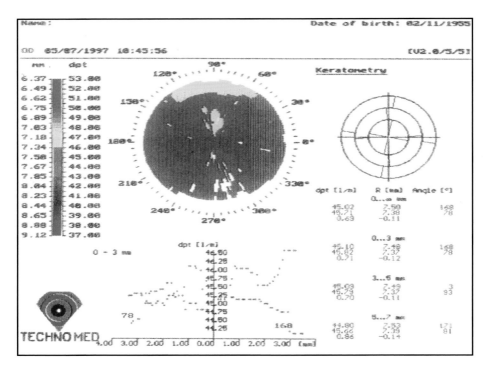

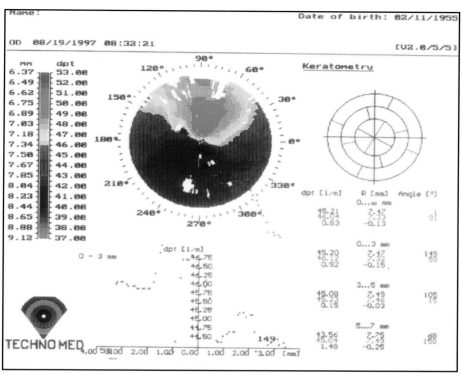

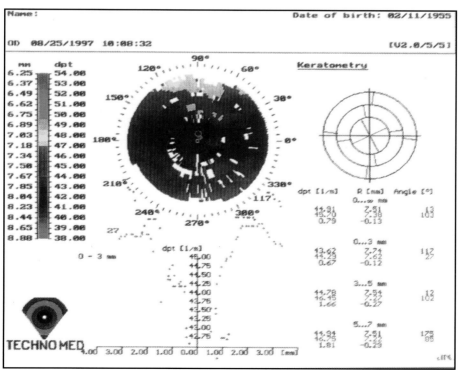

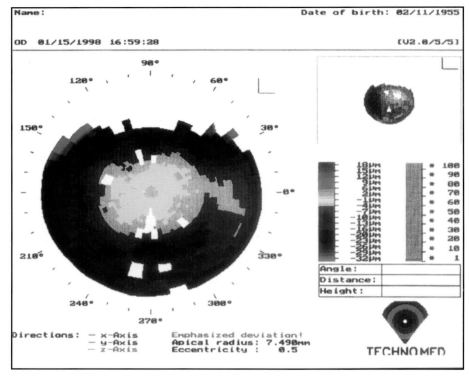

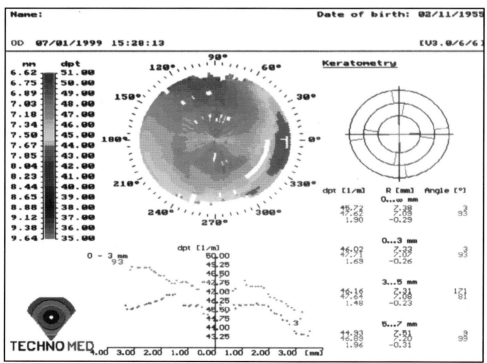

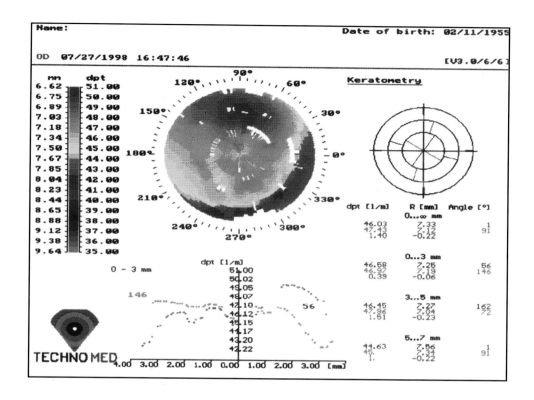

PATIENT EXAMPLE 5

Buttonhole

This 52-year-old woman had a history of rigid gas permeable contact lens use for 35 years, discontinued 1 year prior to workup. Her past eye history included corneal ulcer OU secondary to contact lens overuse and a history of dryness. Her general health was very good. She took no systemic medications. She is left-eye dominant.

Her vision without correction was count fingers at 1 meter OU. Her manifest was -10.75 -1.50 x 177 OD and -10.50 -0.75 x 141 OS. Her manifest vision was 20/20[-2] OU. Manual keratometry was 45.62 @ 172, 47.00 @ 82 OD and 45.75 x 157 x 46.75 @ 67 OS. IOPs and pachymetry were normal. The slit lamp exam was normal with the exception of 1+ SPK OU and diffuse peripheral cortical opacities of the lens OU. The fundus exam was normal OU.

A lengthy discussion regarding risks and benefits ensued and the consent was signed. LASIK OD was performed; and 2 days after LASIK, her vision without correction was 20/25[-2]. LASIK OS was attempted approximately 1 week after OD. A corneal flap was attempted with the ACS microkeratome; however, the flap was quite thin and a buttonhole was noted centrally. It was felt there might have been a loss of suction during the microkeratome pass. On reviewing the videotape, it appeared that there was a stop/start at the beginning of the microkeratome pass. The buttonholed flap was repositioned by lifting and irrigating under the flap, which was followed by a 5-minute wait. The laser treatment was not done.

Two days postoperatively OS, the patient was using Ocuflox (Allergan Pharmaceuticals, Inc, Irvine, Calif) drops qid, FML (Allergan Pharmaceuticals, Inc) drops qid, and Celluvisc (Allergan Pharmaceuticals, Inc, Markham, Ontario) prn. There was a slight irregularity to the epithelium centrally; however, there was no staining with fluorescein. At 1 week, the BCVA OS was 20/20[-2]. At 5 weeks postoperatively, OD VASC was at 20/40[-2] with manifest refraction of -1.25 -0.75 x 75, and enhancement was done OD.

At 3 weeks postoperatively, OS epithelial nests were noticed under the flap around the buttonhole in the visual axis, and there was pooling of fluorescein at the edge of the buttonhole area. Removal of epithelial ingrowth OS was done by lifting and debriding the flap around the buttonhole inside and outside and debriding the bed over and around the button. The flap was then repositioned. Two weeks after removal of epithelial ingrowth OS, the manifest refraction was -8.00 -0.25 x 165, BCVA of 20/25. It was noted that there was haze in a circular pattern outlining the buttonhole with central clearing, no staining with fluorescein.

Five months after the epithelial debridement OS, the manifest refraction was -9.5 -0.75 x 120 with a BCVA of 20/20[-2]. Subepithelial haze was noted around the buttonhole margins. LASIK enhancement was done OS by recutting with a 160 μm depth plate again (no 180 was available). There were no irregularities of the stromal bed and no other complication. The 1-day postoperative vision without correction was 20/30[-3].

At 1.5 years postoperative LASIK OD and 1 year, 2 months postoperative LASIK enhancement OS, VASC OD was 20/30[-3] and 20/25[-1] OS. The manifest refraction was -1.00 sphere OD and -0.25 -0.50 x 50 OS with a BCVA of 20/25[-2] OD and 20/20[-3] OS. The initial buttonhole was still faintly visible, and the patient was very satisfied with her vision for distance and wore readers only for fine print.

In this case, the steep keratometry readings (46.31 D OD and 46.25 D OS) indicate that this patient is at a higher risk for a buttonhole or thin flap. This case further illustrates that epithelial ingrowth may occur at the edges of a buttonhole. Epithelial debridement was done, and BCVA was maintained. When LASIK was again attempted, a successful outcome was obtained. It was felt that a loss of suction in this case might have occurred due to a stop/start during the pass on the initial attempt. Although a deeper depth plate was not available for the retreatment, it may be advisable to use a 180 μ depth plate for steeper corneas and on recuts after thin flaps and buttonholes.

The accompanying photo demonstrates the appearance of the buttonhole at 18 days postoperatively, and one can see epithelial thickening at the edges of the buttonhole. The accompanying maps show preoperative map OS, map following epithelial debridement, and the map postoperative enhancement OS.

(Text and figures reprinted with permission from Gimbel HV, Anderson Penno EE. *LASIK Complications: Prevention and Management.* Thorofare, NJ: SLACK Incorporated, 1999.)

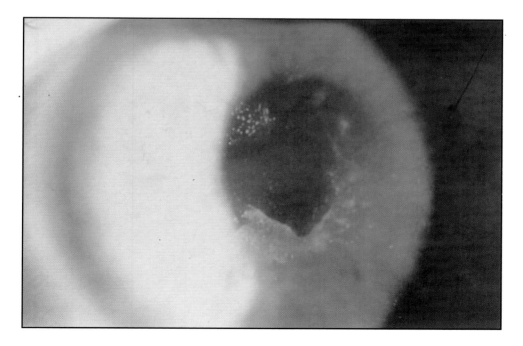

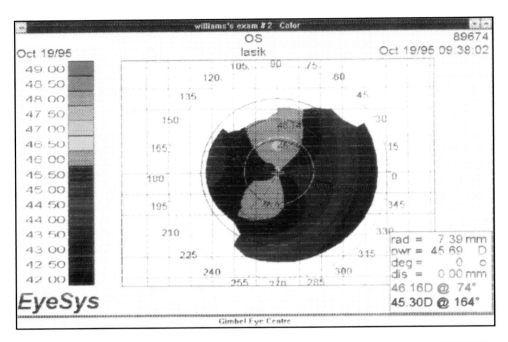

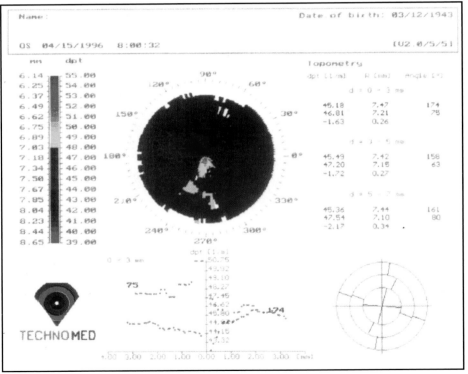

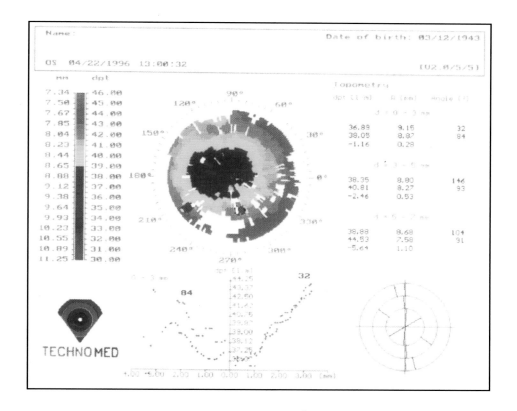

PATIENT EXAMPLE 6

Thin Flap/Inadequate Suction

This 40-year-old man was OS dominant. He stated that his vision OD was never good as a child. His general health was good, and he took no medication. Uncorrected vision was count fingers at 50 cm OU. Manifest refraction was -16.25 -1.75 x 10 with BCVA of 20/20[-3] OD and -17.50 sphere with 20/25 OS. The slit lamp and fundus exams were normal.

As LASIK OD was performed, the IOP was noted to be just barely to the ring of the tonometer. After lifting the flap, it was noted to be thin with some microridges noted near the hinge OD. The ablation was performed. Postoperatively, the flap was in good position. At 1 day postoperative, VASC was 20/70[-1] and manifest refraction was -1.00 -0.75 x 94 with BCVA of 20/40[-3]. The flap was noted to be in good position with trace debris within the flap inferiorly and slightly mottled appearance to the central cornea. The anterior chamber was noted to have trace flare. At 7 months postoperatively LASIK OD, uncorrected vision was 20/400. The manifest refraction was -3.25 -1.25 @ 45 best corrected to 20/30[+2]. The flap was noted to be in good position.

LASIK enhancement was attempted OD. An attempt was made to recut with the microkeratome because of the thin flap after the first surgery; however, the IOP was not adequate to make a new LASIK flap. An attempt was made to dissect the flap, but we were unable to dissect the flap because of adhesions of the flap to the stroma near the hinge.

At a later date, because of the prior difficulty with LASIK, a PRK enhancement was performed OD. Eight months after enhancement, the patient wanted further enhancement OD. The uncorrected vision was 20/80[-2] OD, with a manifest refraction of -3.50 sphere corrected to 20/30[-2]. Slit lamp exam showed no stromal haze centrally and no wrinkles or folding in flap OD.

Basic enhancement was subsequently performed OD with a recut of the flap. VASC OD was 20/50[+2] and manifest refraction was +0.75 -0.50 x 55 best corrected to 20/30[4] months after enhancement.

LASIK OS was then attempted, and there was an incomplete microkeratome pass. The patient complained of pain, and the instrument stopped at about 40% of the travel. The flap was in good position, and no debris was noted. Laser treatment was not performed. LASIK was attempted OS at a later date using the same depth plate and was successful.

At 2 months postoperative, OS uncorrected vision was 20/100[-1]. Manifest refraction was -1.50 -1.25 x 172 with vision of 20/25[-3] OS. The flap was noted to be in good position. The patient was satisfied with his vision OS and did not wish to pursue further treatment at this time.

This is a case in which inadequate suction appears to have resulted in a thin flap. It also points out that the Barraquer tonometer is not a precise instrument, and the surgeon's judgment is needed to decide if the cut should proceed. In this case, the ablation was performed; but in general, ablation should not be performed until a proper depth cut is achieved. These decisions need to be made rather quickly to avoid flap and stromal bed desiccation.

This case also illustrates that in rare cases it may be difficult to dissect the flap for retreatment and also that globe and/or orbital anatomy may predispose to inadequate suction. In this case, poor suction was noted both in the primary and at the time of the first enhancement on the right eye.

On the left eye, the complaint of pain as the microkeratome stopped suggests that the incomplete pass may have been the result of interference from the lids. This is a case in which more than one complication occurred in the same patient.

(Reprinted with permission from Gimbel HV, Anderson Penno EE. *LASIK Complications: Prevention and Management.* Thorofare, NJ: SLACK Incorporated, 1999.)

PATIENT EXAMPLE 7

Free Cap

This patient was a 29-year-old man who was right-eye dominant and had a history of strabismus surgery OS. Soft contact lens wear was stopped 3 years ago due to an allergy to contact lens solution. His general medical health was good, and he was taking no systemic or ocular medications. His uncorrected vision was 20/40 OD and 20/80 OS. The manifest refraction was +5.25 sphere, best corrected to 20/15⁻¹ OD and +6.50 sphere best corrected to 20/30 OS. He was amblyopic OS. Pachymetry was within normal. Keratometry readings were 38.75 @ 16 x 39.00 @ 106 OD, and 38.75 @ 1214 x 39.12 @ 34 OS. The corneal diameters were 12.5 OU, and IOP was within normal. The patient was noted to have no binocularity. The slit lamp exam and fundus exams were normal OU.

LASIK was scheduled to be performed bilaterally. LASIK was performed OS using the Chiron ACS, and a free cap was created. The laser ablation was performed, and the cap was replaced. The cap diameter was 7.75 mm, and the hyperopic ablation diameter was 5.5 mm with a transition zone of 7.5 mm. Surgery OD was postponed pending stabilization of OS.

At 1 day postoperative, vision OS without correction was 20/50⁺² and corrected was 20/30⁻². There was mild stromal edema, and no wrinkles or folds were noted in the flap. The interface was clean, and there was mild staining at the incision site, but no gaps were noted.

The patient was warned of the increased risk for free cap OD; however, LASIK OD was subsequently performed using the same keratome without complications. At 11 months postoperative LASIK OU, the patient stated that his vision was good for distance, blurry for near. He had no other complaints. His uncorrected vision was 20/20 OD and 20/30 OS. Cycloplegic refraction showed +3.75 -0.50 x 155 OD and +4.25 -0.50 x 8 OS. BCVA was 20/25⁺² OD and 20/30 OS. Manual keratometry showed 40.00 @ 3 x 41.37 @ 93 OD and 40.75 @ 176 x 41.87 @ 86 OS. IOPs were normal. A slit lamp exam revealed trace SPK OD with fine microstriation at the hinge on retroillumination OD and moderate fibrosis at the cap incision at 1 o'clock with moderate fibrosis along the cap incision extending from 4 to 9 o'clock. There were no wrinkles or folds in the flap.

At the time of enhancement OS, some epithelial ingrowth was noted at the 4 o'clock position. This was removed after the cap was turned. It was also noted that the inferotemporal edge of the cap was quite thin. At 2 weeks after the enhancement OS, there was noted to be epithelial ingrowth that appeared to be extending. At 1 month postoperative, it was felt that because the ingrowth was not pearl colored or resulting in a melt, removal should be scheduled on a nonurgent basis.

At 2 months postoperative, epithelial ingrowth was noted to be from 4 to 10 o'clock about 1 to 2 mm wide peripherally and appeared as islands under the flap. The ingrowth was not in the visual axis, and the flap was not necrotic. Due to patient scheduling, the enhancement was scheduled for 5 months after the enhancement surgery OS.

At 5 months post-enhancement OS, UVCA was 20/25^{+2} OD and 20/50^{+2} OS. A cycloplegic refraction OS was +2.00 -1.25 x 30, best corrected to 20/40. The slit lamp exam revealed a ring of pigment deposition in the mid-periphery of the flap with traces centrally, mild fibrosis at the flap incision OD, and moderate haze and fibrosis along the incision at 3 o'clock with mild mid-peripheral haze.

The cap was turned, and removal of epithelial ingrowth was performed. A contact lens was placed. At 1 day postoperatively, VASC was 20/40^{-3} OS. Cap margins were visible. There was an area of loose epithelium along the inferior edge of the cap with no obvious debris in the interface. There was a contact lens in place. At the third postoperative day, the contact lens was removed, and there were small areas of stain over one area of loose epithelium; however, the epithelium appeared intact.

Over the course of the following year he developed epithelial ingrowth one more time. This was removed and has not recurred to date. He continues to have UCVA 20/40^{-2} with no improvement on refraction.

The accompanying photo was taken after the first enhancement. The iron line corresponds to the hyperopic ablation pattern. The fibrosis at the edges and epithelial ingrowth in this case were related to hyperopic correction and not free cap. Sometimes, the ablation will spill outside the bed if slightly decentered, which may be a risk factor for epithelial ingrowth. In this case the cap diameter was 7.75 mm, and the transition zone was 7.5 mm. Thin edges should also be shielded with a Chayet drain, so epithelium and stroma are not ablated.

In this case, the cap was replaced without the use of sutures and remained in place after both the primary and enhancement surgeries, demonstrating that sutures are not necessarily indicated when a free cap is obtained. Hyperopic LASIK is now only performed after 9.5 to 10.0 mm flaps are obtained with the Hansatome and an optical zone of 5.5 mm transitioning to 9.0 mm is used. Higher corrections and less regression are obtained.

(Text and figure reprinted with permission from Gimbel HV, Anderson Penno EE. *LASIK Complications: Prevention and Management.* Thorofare, NJ: SLACK Incorporated, 1999.)

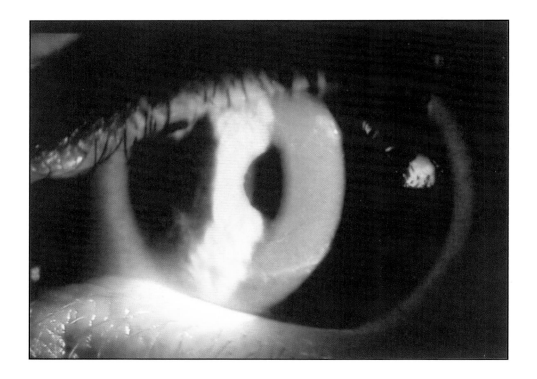

PATIENT EXAMPLE 8

Flap Shrinkage

This 26-year-old man had no previous medical or ocular problems and was on no medications. His uncorrected vision was 20/70⁻¹ OD and 20/80⁻¹ OS. The cycloplegic refraction revealed +1.75 -3.50 x 173 corrected to 20/15⁻¹ OD and +3.25 -4.00 x 176 OS corrected to 20/15⁻² OS. Pachymetry was within normal OU. Manual keratometry was 39.87 @ 174 x 42.37 @ 84 OD and 39.37 @ 3 x 42.62 @ 93 OS. Corneal diameters were 11.50 mm OD and 12.00 mm OS. IOPs were within normal OU. Pupils measured 6.00 mm in bright light and 7.50 mm in dim lighting OU. Slit lamp exam and dilated fundus exam were within normal.

LASIK was performed OU. The epithelium was unusually loose considering his age, and it abraded from the microkeratome pass OD more so than OS. After the laser ablation OD, the corneal flap was moistened and replaced in the original position using forceps so as not to further disturb the epithelium. Gentle irrigation was done under the flap using a 30-gauge cannula. An attempt was made to reposition the loose epithelium, but it was too torn and stretched to approximate exactly. The flap was inspected for wrinkles or debris, and fluid was dried from the edges. Verification of the position using the gentian violet marks was done. While trying to manage the epithelial problem, the flap contracted, leaving a wide gutter. It was decided to suture the flap because of this and the loose epithelium. Eight 10-0 sutures were used to keep the flap in position. Further irrigation under the flap was done to remove a particle of lint, and the flap was again inspected for wrinkles and debris. OS simply required a soft contact lens due to poor epithelial adherence.

By the second postoperative day, the contacts were removed OU. The slit lamp exam found the epithelium intact with small infiltrates centrally OS. There was still a large defect inferior temporally OD, which developed as soon as the contact lens was removed. Loose epithelium was debrided, and a second bandage lens was instilled OD. On the third postoperative day, the right eye showed 1+ conjunctival injection, no infiltrates, and the contact lens was in place. There was still a defect noted. The left eye showed epithelial filaments at the nasal border of the pupil. On the fourth postoperative day, the contact was removed OD. The epithelium OD showed a speckled appearance but was intact.

At 1 month postoperatively, the sutures were removed OD. The uncorrected vision at the 1-month postoperative visit was 20/80⁻¹ OD and 20/20⁻¹ OS. BCVA was 20/40 OD and 20/15 OS. An enhancement was done due to under-response OD. Again, loose epithelium was noted intraoperatively. On the first postoperative day, there was noted to be a wide central corneal abrasion with some peripheral epithelial tags. The patient was taken to the operating room, the epithelium was smoothed, and the epithelial tags were removed. A soft contact lens was then instilled.

At 1 week postoperatively, the epithelium had healed, and the uncorrected vision OD was 20/40. At 3 weeks postoperatively, uncorrected vision was 20/40 OD, refraction +1.00 -3.50 x 180, with vision correctable to 20/30⁻. Subsequent enhancements were performed for residual hyperopic astigmatism without difficulty. His final UCVA was 20/20[3] with a manifest refraction of plano -0.25 x 175 corrected to 20/20.

This patient demonstrates that epithelial adherence will vary between patients; however, if loose epithelium is encountered on the first eye, it is likely to be encountered on the second eye. Epithelial complications will not often pose a long-term problem but can significantly prolong postoperative discomfort and delay recovery of vision. Because many patients who choose to have LASIK have busy schedules and only plan to take a day or two off work, these delays can be a significant inconvenience. The accompanying photograph demonstrates the sutures that were used to stretch the flap back into position after encountering flap shrinkage intraoperatively.

(Text and figure reprinted with permission from Gimbel HV, Anderson Penno EE. *LASIK Complications: Prevention and Management.* Thorofare, NJ: SLACK Incorporated, 1999.)

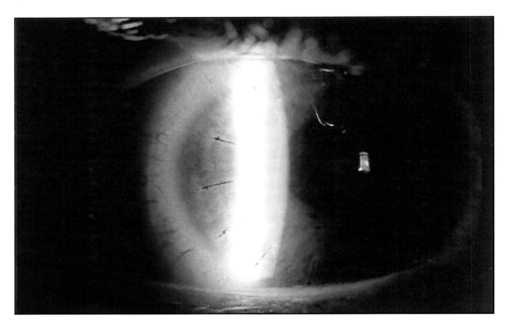

Epithelial Disruption/LASIK Attempt

This 47-year-old man had no eye problems but had a history of Crohn's disease. Medications were vitamins B12, C, and E. Vision without correction was 20/400 OU. The manifest refraction was -6.25 -1.00 @ 35 corrected to 20/15^{-1} OD and -6.50 -0.50 @ 105 corrected to 20/15^{-3} OS. Manual keratometry readings were 41.12 @ 17 x 42.12 @ 107 and 41.50 @ 153 x 42.25 @ 63. The slit lamp exam revealed 1+ NS OU and was otherwise normal.

LASIK OS using the Hansatome resulted in an area of loose epithelium, but the epithelium was not torn. A contact lens was placed for 24 hours. LASIK OD resulted in denuded epithelium with no flap created. The reason this happened was inattention to the preoperative check of the Hansatome. The motor shaft did not engage the slot in the blade holder and, therefore, did not move the blade as the microkeratome made its pass across the eye. The stationary blade did, however, abrade much of the epithelium in the area of the cornea where the flap should have been cut. The epithelium was denuded except for an area midpupil to superior mid-periphery. The stroma was not cut. The abraded epithelium was replaced as much as possible, and a contact lens was placed (see Figure 5-18). The patient was maintained on tobramycin/dexamethasone, and the contact lens was removed on the fourth postoperative day. By 2 weeks postoperatively, VA OD returned to 20/20 with a manifest of -6.50 -0.50 @ 27. Uncorrected vision OS was 20/25^{-3} with manifest of +0.75 -0.50 @ 45.

Six weeks after the LASIK attempt OD, the flap was recut successfully and laser ablation was done. Loose epithelium was noted intraoperatively, and a contact lens was placed. At 2 days postoperatively, the bandage lens was in place. The patient complained of excessive tearing. The epithelium was intact but there was an irregularity at the flap margin. Tobramycin/dexamethasone ointment was instilled and, because of the discomfort, the contact lens was removed and an eye patch was applied. The patient was checked daily, and the patch was reapplied. On the fourth postoperative day, the irregularity remained; however, there was no uptake of fluorescein, and the patch was discontinued. The patient was continued on tobramycin/dexamethasone and artificial tears.

At 3 months postoperative LASIK OD, and 4.5 months postoperative LASIK OS, VASC was 20/80-2 OD and 20/20 OS. Manifest refraction revealed -1.00 -0.50 x 100 best corrected to 20/25^{+2} OD, and plano -0.25 x 61 best corrected to 20/20 OS.

An enhancement was performed OD, and again a contact lens was placed for loose epithelium. The contact lens was necessary for 10 days postoperatively. The flap remained in good position. At 1 month post-enhancement OD, VASC was 20/30^{-3}, and manifest refraction was +0.75 sphere with best-corrected vision of 20/20. The flap was in good position, and it was noted that there was a tiny patch of epithelial ingrowth at the 4 o'clock position at the flap edge. The patient stated that although the vision OD was not "super sharp," it was satisfactory and the decision was made to continue close follow-up both with regard to refraction and the tiny patch of epithelial ingrowth. A year after enhancement, the UCVA was 20/20- [2] with no improvement with manifest refraction. The patient was satisfied with his vision.

This is an example in which inattention to the preoperative check of the Hansatome occurred, and it was not noted prior to proceeding that the blade was not engaged. This highlights the importance of visual verification that all parts are moving appropriately and freely (as outlined in Chapter 3). In addition to the prolonged postoperative discomfort and blurred vision, epithelial complications may pose a risk for epithelial ingrowth, as occurred in this patient. This example also illustrates that some patients may be prone to loose epithelium even in the absence of equipment malfunction. This patient's eye is pictured in Figure 5-18. In most cases, a contact lens can be placed until the epithelium has healed; however, occasionally, as occurred in this patient, a pressure patch may be required to ensure patient comfort. Patches should be applied only when the patient cannot tolerate a contact lens, and great care should be used when placing the patch as there may be a risk of flap dislocation, especially if applied on the day of surgery.

(Reprinted with permission from Gimbel HV, Anderson Penno EE. *LASIK Complications: Prevention and Management.* Thorofare, NJ: SLACK Incorporated, 1999.)

PATIENT EXAMPLE 10

Flap Repositioning

This was a 41-year-old presbyopic woman. She had no past eye problems, was in good medical health, was taking no medications, and was right-eye dominant. Uncorrected vision was count fingers at 3 meters OU. Cycloplegic refraction was -10.75 -1.25 x 17, with vision 20/20· 3 OD and -10.75 -2.25 x 163, vision 20/20+2 OS. Pachymetry was 0.519 µ OD and 0.522 µ OS. Manual keratometry was 45.12 @ 6 x 46.75 @ 96 OD and 44.12 @ 166 x 46.37 @ 76 OS. Corneal diameters were 11 mm. Slit lamp exam was notable for trace SPK and blepharitis OU with trace nuclear sclerosis OU. Fundus exam was within normal OU.

LASIK OS was done without complications using the Chiron ACS. The flap was in good position at the postoperative check. At 1 day postoperative, the patient stated that OS felt a bit sore and vision was improved but still blurry. VASC was 20/80; and on slit lamp exam, it was noted that there was reduced tear break-up time. There was a 1+ subconjunctival hemorrhage superior nasally, there were wrinkles and multiple wrinkling at the hinge area with mild epithelial edema, trace SPK, slight inferior decentration of the flap with a gap visible superiorly, and staining at the superior flap incision.

The patient was taken back to the OR on the first postoperative day for repositioning. The flap was found to be rotated inferiorly approximately 0.5 to 1 mm. Some crescent wrinkles were noted inferior nasally from the hinge. The flap was elevated with the irrigation cannula, and excess epithelium superiorly was excised. The flap was turned, and a spatula was used to scrape and stretch the flap near the hinge to stretch out the wrinkles. This did not seem to help, because there were ridges of the flap stroma that were not smoothed out. The stromal bed was wiped with a Paton spatula, particularly near the edges to remove the overlying epithelium. The flap was repositioned. There were still deep wrinkles in the epithelium. It was felt that these may be persistent stromal wrinkles. The flap was stretched by stroking from the hinge outward. When good flap position was verified, a gentian violet mark was made. The flap was lifted once more to recontour and then was gently repositioned. Fluid was then expressed with the spatula. The edges were dried. After 8 minutes, Alcaine (Alcon, Ft. Worth, Tex), Ocuflox, and an 8.8 Acuvue contact lens (Johnson & Johnson Vision Products Inc, Jacksonville, Fla) was applied.

The patient was rechecked 30 minutes postoperatively, and it was found that the flap was decentered again under the contact lens. The patient was taken back to the OR, and the flap was repositioned again after the bed and flap were cleaned. To avoid further flap slippage, a 10-0 nylon Guimaraes bra suture was placed in a cross fashion across the flap. A contact lens was then re-applied, and Ocuflox, tobramycin/dexamethasone, and Cyclogyl (Alcon, Fort Worth, Tex) were applied.

The patient was examined the following morning, and the flap was again shifted. The patient was brought back to the OR for the third repositioning. The 10-0 nylon Guimaraes bra suture was removed, and the LASIK flap was lifted. The Paton spatula was used to brush and straighten the flap. The flap was floated back into position, and the edges were dried with a Merocel sponge. A Katena axis marker (Katena Product, Inc, Denville, NJ) coated with gentian violet was used to make three orientation marks temporally. A 10-0 nylon bra suture was again placed more tightly, and an eye patch was placed. On the 45-minute postoperative recheck, the flap was in good position.

On the first postoperative day after the third flap repositioning, the patch was removed and the flap was in good position. Epithelial defects had healed, the suture was removed, and the eye was repatched. On the second postoperative day, there was mild epithelial edema over the flap, the flap was in good position, and there was a small epithelial defect noted. The flap was in good position. The patch was to be left on for another 24 hours.

LASIK OD was performed without complications. However, on the first check at 30 minutes postoperatively, it was noted that in this eye the flap was shifted inferiorly. A same-day repositioning was performed. Gentle irrigation under the flap was performed. The flap was moistened and replaced to the original position. The flap was inspected for wrinkles and debris, and fluid was dried from the edges, Ocuflox drops were instilled, and a pressure patch was applied. The eye was inspected 30 minutes postoperatively, and the flap was in good position.

After the second postoperative check (approximately 30 minutes after the first postoperative check), it was noted that the flap had again shifted. The patient was brought back to the operating room, and the eye was prepped in the usual manner. The corneal flap was moistened and replaced in the original position. Gentle irrigation was done under the flap and fluid dried from the edges. After waiting 10 minutes and 7 seconds, Ocuflox drops and Muro 128 drops (Bausch & Lomb, St. Louis, Mo) were instilled. After waiting approximately 5 minutes, the flap was noted to be in good position. The patient remained in the operating room chair for approximately 45 minutes. The flap was rechecked and noted to be in good position. Further Muro 128 drops were instilled and the patient was taken to the recovery room in good condition.

Again, at the 30-minute check, it was noted again that the flap had shifted. The patient was brought back to the laser suite, and again prepped in the usual manner. The flap was moistened and replaced in the original position. Gentle irrigation was done under the flap using a 30-gauge cannula. Proparacaine hydrochloride drops were instilled, and a Guimaraes bra suture was placed to keep the flap in place. Pentamycetin (Sabex, Boucherville, Quebec) ointment and an eye patch were applied. After the third repositioning, the patch was removed approximately 30 minutes later, and the flap was in good position.

On the first postoperative day, it was noted that the flap was still in good position, the suture was intact, but there was a central 3.5-mm epithelial defect. On the second postoperative day, the suture was removed; and at the 4-day postoperative visit OD, the flap remained in place and the epithelial defect was closed.

In both eyes, persistent superficial punctate keratopathy and 1 to 2+ flap edema was encountered. There was mild cellular AC reaction accompanying these findings. The patient had been on tobramycin/dexamethasone and Ocuflox drops with

Pentamycetin ointment at bedtime. The Pentamycetin ointment and tobramycin/dexamethasone were discontinued, and the patient was switched to FML and Celluvisc; however, the epithelial keratitis continued. At 1 month postoperatively, the steroid was discontinued and preservative-free artificial tears were continued. The VASC was 20/40[+2] OD and 20/70 OS. The manifest refraction at that time was -1.25 -1.00 x 25, BCVA 20/25[-3] OD and -1.25 -100 x 105 BCVA 20/40[-2] OS. The continued loss of BCVA was attributed to continued diffuse SPK OU and filamentary keratitis.

At 8 months postoperatively OD and 9 months postoperatively OS, VASC was 20/60 OD and 20/30[-1] OS with a manifest of -0.75 -1.00 x 89 corrected to 20/40 OD and -0.25 -0.75 x 106 corrected to 20/25[-2] OS. Diffuse SPK was noted OD, and mild blepharitis was noted OU. The patient was advised to continue preservative-free lubricants and begin warm compresses for blepharitis. Enhancements were not planned at this time.

Of note was that the striae test was done on both eyes on all of the repositionings, and in spite of apparently good adherence, the flap continued to dislocate. Also of note was that this surgery was done prior to the use of moisture chambers as a routine postoperatively. In retrospect, it was also noted that this patient's eyes were somewhat exophthalmic with some upper eyelid retraction. This is now recognized as a risk factor in LASIK surgery. Possibly, with a superior hinge, this patient would not have had any dislocations.

This case further illustrates the importance of careful examination preoperatively, with careful notation of lid retraction, lagophthalmos, and pre-existing SPK. If lagophthalmos or other lid or orbital abnormalities are noted on the preoperative exam, the patient may be at risk for complications such as those encountered in this case.

(Reprinted with permission from Gimbel HV, Anderson Penno EE. *LASIK Complications: Prevention and Management*. Thorofare, NJ: SLACK Incorporated, 1999.)

PATIENT EXAMPLE 11

LASIK Flap Repositioning and Suturing

This patient was a 51-year-old man who did not wear contact lenses. He was left-eye dominant and had no medical health conditions. He took no medications and had no previous eye problems. Uncorrected vision was count fingers at 1.5 meters OU. The manifest refraction was -8.50 -1.00 x 136 with vision of 20/20 [1] OD and -7.50 -0.75 x 96 with vision of 20/15 [1] OS. Pachymetry was within normal. Manual keratometry showed 46.75 @ 168 x 47.75 @ 78 OD and 47.00 @ 120 x 48.12 @ 30 OS. Corneal diameters were 10.75 mm OU, and slit lamp exam and fundus exam were normal OU.

Primary LASIK was done OU and proceeded without complications. At 5 months postoperative LASIK OU, VASC was 20/60 [2] with a manifest refraction of -1.00 - 0.75 x 101 and vision of 20/15 OD, and VASC of 20/100 with a manifest of -1.75 - 0.50 x 149 and vision of 20/15 [3] OS.

The flaps were in good position at the postoperative visit. Enhancement was done OS. There was poor epithelial adherence, so a contact lens was placed, and surgery was canceled OD. At the 30-minute postoperative slit lamp exam, the flap was in good position, and the contact lens was in place. At 1 day postoperatively, the contact lens was removed, and the flap was noted to be shifted inferiorly with numerous striae. The patient was taken back to the operating room for repositioning and suturing. Intraoperatively, the flap was noted to be shifted inferiorly with exposure of approximately one-half of the bed. Epithelium was cleared from the bed and the edges of the flap. The flap was repositioned and then sutured in place with interrupted 10-0 nylon sutures.

Six days postoperatively, three sutures were removed because they were partially exposed. The interface was noted to be clean. There was an epithelial filament inferior nasally that was removed. The patient was instructed to return in 1 week.

At 2 weeks, all sutures were removed, and the patient was instructed to use tobramycin/dexamethasone (tid). Uncorrected vision at that visit was 20/200 with manifest refraction -1.00 -1.50 x 125 and correction to 20/20 OS. At 3 months following flap repositioning, VASC was 20/20 OS with a manifest of +0.50 -0.25 x 130 with a BCVA of 20/15 [2]. The corneal exam revealed fine fibrosis at the incision and suture sites. The flap was in good position with no wrinkles or folds. At the 3-month follow-up examination, his UCVA was 20/20 with a manifest refraction of +0.50 - 0.25 x 130 corrected to 20/15 [2]. The patient was pleased with his vision.

The average keratometry readings in this case were 47.25 D OD and 47.56 D OS. In spite of these steep corneas, there were no thin flap or buttonhole complications. This emphasizes that the occurrence of thin flaps or buttonholes is likely due to a variety of factors, and steep corneas pose an increased risk but not a contraindication to LASIK surgery. It is likely that poor epithelial adherence may indicate a higher risk for poor flap adherence on the basis of fluid dynamics. While some surgeons routinely place a contact lens postoperatively, others feel that placing a contact lens may be a risk for flap shifting. However, in some cases, it is necessary for patient comfort, and a contact lens is, in most cases, preferable to a pressure patch. The decision as to whether or not to use sutures after flap repositioning will depend on epithelial adherence and flap adherence. Again, with proper management (as in this case), the outcome is excellent, and there is no loss of BCVA.

The photograph shows the flap sutures in place at day 1 postoperatively.

(Text and figures reprinted with permission from Gimbel HV, Anderson Penno EE. *LASIK Complications: Prevention and Management.* Thorofare, NJ: SLACK Incorporated, 1999.)

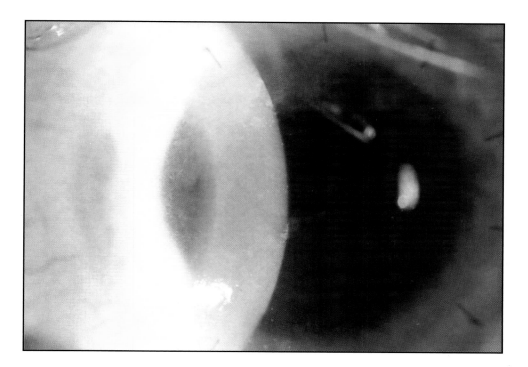

PATIENT EXAMPLE 12

Flap Repositioning

This was a 47-year-old woman with a history of wearing gas permeable lenses for 30 years. She had tried monovision with no problems previously. She had no other ocular problems. She had a history of asthma and was taking Premarin Slow (Wyeth-Ayerst Canada Inc. St. Laurent, Quebec) bid. Uncorrected vision was 20/400 OU. Her manifest refraction was -6.25 -0.50 x 166 with vision of 20/20 OD and -6.50 -0.75 x 178 with 20/20 OS. Pachymetry was normal. Manual keratometry was 45.25 @ 172 x 47.50 @ 82 OD and 45.50 @ 5 x 47.12 @ 95 OS. Corneal diameters were 11.50 OU. Slit lamp exam showed trace cortical lens changes OU. Fundus exam was normal.

The patient elected to proceed with LASIK with monovision for OS. LASIK was performed OU using the ACS. There were no intraoperative complications in either eye. The patient called shortly after surgery stating that vision was very poor in her left eye compared to the right and that the left eye was very foggy for near and distance. She was concerned about the flap. She did not complain of any discomfort. The flap was noted to be shifted, and the patient was brought back to the operating room 4 hours postoperative. Gentle irrigation under the flap was used and the corneal flap was then moistened and replaced into the original position using BSS to float it into position. The interface was inspected, and verification of proper positioning was done. Adherence was also verified.

At 1 day postoperatively, the patient stated that the vision was quite "waxy." Her uncorrected vision OD was 20/40- 3, pinholed to 20/15- 3. VASC OS was 20/70 pinholed to 20/40- 2. Slit lamp exam revealed no wrinkles or folds in the flap with the inferior aspect of the flap showing 1+ epithelial irregularity and mild stromal edema OD. Slit lamp exam OS revealed no wrinkles or folds in the flap, 2+ diffuse SPK, moderate stromal edema along the flap incision, and moderate epithelial irregularity.

At 2 days postoperatively, vision without correction was 20/30- 2 OD. Uncorrected vision OS was 20/60- 2 with a manifest refraction of -1.00 -1.25 x 4 and vision of 20/25- 3. At the slit lamp, it was noted that there was some epithelial edema at the edge of the flap.

At 5 weeks postoperatively, her UCVA was 20/25+ OD and 20/100 OS with a manifest refraction of -0.25 sphere with 20/20 OD and -1.75 sphere with 20/20 OS (targeted for monovision). The flap was noted to be in good position OU.

Photographs of this patient are shown in Figures 5-11a and b. This example illustrates that any patient who complains that the vision becomes foggy postoperatively regardless of whether or not there is discomfort should have a slit lamp exam. In this case, there was no accompanying discomfort. There was no clear cause for flap shifting in this case, although it is possible that the patient inadvertently rubbed her eye. This complication also occurred before we began using the moisture chamber routinely.

(Reprinted with permission from Gimbel HV, Anderson Penno EE. *LASIK Complications: Prevention and Management.* Thorofare, NJ: SLACK Incorporated, 1999.)

PATIENT EXAMPLE 13

Flap Repositioning

This 41-year-old man had no previous eye problems, was right-eye dominant, in good medical health, and took no medications. Uncorrected vision was count fingers at 1 meter OD and count fingers at 50 cm OS. Cycloplegic refraction revealed -13.00 -0.50 x 100 corrected to 20/20 OD and -12.25 -0.75 x 80 corrected to 20/20 OS. Pachymetry was within normal. Manual keratometry was 40.87 @ 160 x 41.25 @ 70 OD, and 40.75 @ 30 x 41.25 @ 120 OS. Corneal diameters were 12 mm OU. Slit lamp and funduscopic exams were within normal.

LASIK was performed OU without complications. The patient was seen at the 3 day postoperative visit. VASC was 20/25[-2] OD with a manifest refraction of -0.75 -0.50 x 105 with best-corrected vision of 20/20[-1]. Vision OS was 20/125, and the manifest revealed -2.00 -1.00 x 60 best corrected to 20/100[-1]. A slit lamp exam revealed intact flap in good position OD and marked central wrinkling of the flap OS.

The patient was brought back to the operating room, and the flap was noted to be shifted inferior-temporally with moderate striae. The flap was turned, and epithelium growing over the flap edge was removed. The epithelial growth on the bed was also removed, and the flap was repositioned. The edges were inspected for symmetry. Ten 10-0 nylon interrupted sutures were placed, and a bandage contact lens was placed. The sutures were removed on the third postoperative day.

Wrinkles reappeared, and resuturing was done 9 days later. The flap was resutured with 10-0 nylon. At 1-week post-enhancement, VASC was 20/30[-2], manifest refraction was -0.75 -0.50 x 150 with vision of 20/20[-3]. The slit lamp exam revealed the flap to be in good position, with no loose sutures or epithelial ingrowth or wrinkles. This patient was noted to be somewhat exophthalmic on follow-up exams.

The sutures were removed at the 6-week visit OS, and vision at that time was 20/25[-3] uncorrected. BCVA was 20/15[-3] with -0.75 -0.25 x 5 OS.

This case demonstrated that sutures need to be left for more than 3 days to keep wrinkles stretched out until fibrosis occurs. This patient's left eye is pictured in Figure 6-5. This patient was also noted to be somewhat exophthalmic on follow-up exams, which may have been a risk factor for a shifted flap. BCVA was preserved at the 6-week visit after the second resuturing demonstrating that with proper management a satisfactory result can be obtained.

(Reprinted with permission from Gimbel HV, Anderson Penno EE. *LASIK Complications: Prevention and Management.* Thorofare, NJ: SLACK Incorporated, 1999.)

PATIENT EXAMPLE 14

Thin Flap/Debris Under Flap

This was a 52-year-old man with no previous eye problems and in good medical health. His vision without correction was count fingers at 2 meters OU, and his manifest vision was -12.00 -2.75 x 14 best corrected to 20/20^{-2} OD and -12.00 -1.25 x 155 best corrected 20/20^{-3} OS. Pachymetry was 0.441 mm OD and 0.439 mm OS. Manual keratometry was 45.00 10 x 46.75 @ 100 OD and 45.62 @ 170 x 47.00 @ 80 OS. Corneal diameters were 12 mm OU. Slit lamp exam revealed trace NS OU, and funduscopic exams were normal OU.

LASIK was done OS without complication, and LASIK OD was attempted; however, an extremely thin flap was obtained. There was a 2.5 to 3 mm central thinning in the flap, and laser ablation was not performed. At 1 day postoperative, the slit lamp exam showed mild epithelial haze centrally with an area of loose epithelium centrally, which was removed and a contact lens was then applied. At 1 week postoperatively, manifest refraction was -12.00 -1.75 x 26 OD with vision of 20/30. At 2 months postoperatively, vision pinholed to 20/25^{-2} OD. At slit lamp exam, the edges of the thin area in the flap OD were noted.

A second attempt at LASIK was done OD at 4 months postoperatively. There was noted to be a slight central epithelial pucker in a radial pattern. At 2 months postoperatively, VASC was 20/20 OD with manifest of +0.25 sphere, best corrected 20/15^{-2} OD.

An enhancement was necessary OS, and there was a small foreign body noted at the nasal edge of the flap OS following uncomplicated LASIK enhancement OS. He was taken back to the laser suite for irrigation. After the first irrigation, a slit lamp exam was performed, and it was noted that the foreign body had moved under a gentian violet mark. The patient was taken back to the laser suite for irrigation a second time. A contact lens was then placed OS for some epithelial disruptions superiorly.

At 2 months post-enhancement, VASC was 20/30 OS, and manifest was -0.50 -0.50 x 80 with vision correctable to 20/20^{-3} OS. Interestingly, the patient presented approximately 4 months post-enhancement with pain and blurriness OS. There was an epithelial disruption centrally that appeared to be herpes simplex keratitis. The patient was placed on Viroptic (Burroughs Wellcome Co, Research Triangle Park, NC). After improvement was noted, he returned to his primary care doctor for follow-up care.

The average keratometry readings in this case were 45.88 D OD and 46.31 D OS. The steepness of the cornea OD was not likely the only reason for the thin central area that resulted in the first failed attempt at LASIK. The suction and raised IOP may have been less OD than OS. Of note is that on the successful second attempt, slight epithelial pucker was noted reflecting the Bowman's membrane scar seen on slit lamp exam from the previous thin flap. This case also demonstrates that, with proper management, the final UCVA was excellent and the BCVA improved.

Similarly, the debris that was noted in the interface OS was easily managed with no loss of BCVA. The development of herpes simplex keratitis was not related to surgery but highlights the fact that the surgeon must be aware of all concurrent ophthalmic problems and is responsible for either management or referral for appropriate management of nonsurgical problems.

In the first photograph, you can see the slight scar that can occur at the edge of a thin flap ablation. This scar is due to a partial cut into the membrane even if the epithelium is not broken. It is not a through-and-through buttonhole but is, in fact, a partial buttonhole of Bowman's. Subsequently, one may get a bit of haze, as demonstrated here. The second photograph illustrates the keratitis that was felt to be Herpes simplex at 4 months post-enhancement surgery OS.

(Text and figures reprinted with permission from Gimbel HV, Anderson Penno EE. *LASIK Complications: Prevention and Management.* Thorofare, NJ: SLACK Incorporated, 1999.)

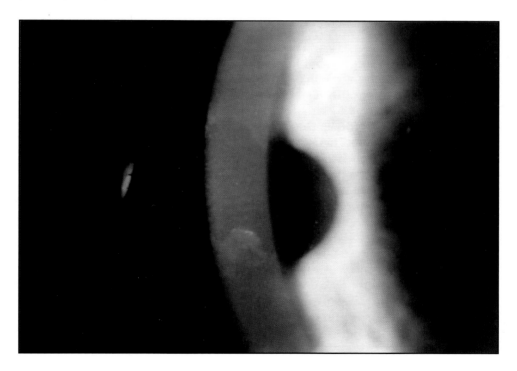

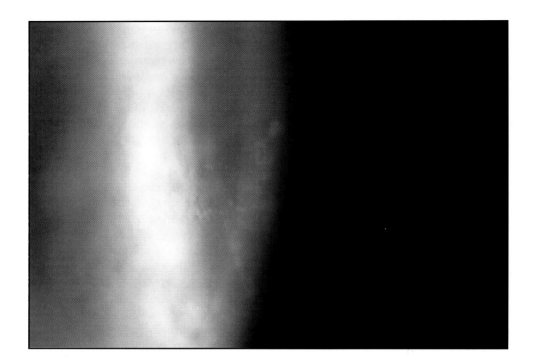

PATIENT EXAMPLE 15

Epithelial Ingrowth

This was a 34-year-old man who was 1 month postoperative LASIK OD and 3 months postoperative LASIK OS, both done elsewhere, who came for a second opinion. His uncorrected vision was 20/30 OD and 20/15 OS. The manifest refraction was +1.50 -1.75 x 32 best corrected to 20/15⁻¹ OD and plano -0.50 to 20/15 OS. It was noted that the mires were distorted OD, and there was an area of lipid appearance with haze nasally. This covered about a 1.7-mm area 1 mm from the visual axis. It was felt that this was epithelial ingrowth. The patient returned to his original ophthalmologist for debridement of the epithelial ingrowth. At 6 weeks post-debridement, the patient's visual acuity without correction was 20/15⁻¹ with a manifest refraction of plano -0.25 x 180 (corrected to 20/15).

There were no obvious risk factors for epithelial ingrowth in this case, such as poor flap adhesion, epithelial abrasion, flap misalignment, or buttonhole at the time of surgery that could be ascertained from the medical record.

This case demonstrated the loss of visual acuity (uncorrected) and irregular astigmatism (distorted keratometry mires) that can result from epithelial ingrowth. This patient recovered excellent uncorrected acuity after debridement of the epithelial ingrowth. Figure 7-2b is a photograph of this case prior to debridement.

(Reprinted with permission from Gimbel HV, Anderson Penno EE. *LASIK Complications: Prevention and Management.* Thorofare, NJ: SLACK Incorporated, 1999.)

PATIENT EXAMPLE 16

Epithelial Ingrowth Resulting in a Stromal Melt

This 44-year-old male underwent primary LASIK for myopic astigmatism OU. He was in good medical health, took no medications, and had no known drug allergies. The manifest refraction was -2.50 sphere corrected to 20/20+2 vision OD and -2.00 -0.50 x 112 corrected to 20/15- 1 vision OS prior to surgery. The surgery on the left eye was unremarkable, but the right eye had an area of loose epithelium. This was smoothed back into position at the conclusion of the LASIK and a contact lens was placed.

On postoperative day 1, the UCVA was 20/25- 2 pinholed to 20/20 OD. The contact lens had fallen out overnight. The flap was well-positioned, but there was an epithelial defect and looseness temporally from 7 to 11 o'clock measuring 6.0 mm by 3.0 mm, as well as a tag of loose epithelium. The left eye had an UCVA of 20/15- 1, and slit lamp examination was unremarkable.The patient was taken back to the operating room and the tag of loose epithelium was removed.

On the fifth postoperative day, the UCVA OD was 20/20- 1. Epithelial irregularity was noted from 7 to 11 o'clock with some localized stromal edema. Prednisolone acetate 6 times a day was started in addition to the Ocuflox. By the second week, all eye medications had been discontinued and the UCVA OD was 20/20- 1 with a manifest refraction of -0.50 sphere corrected to 20/20. The epithelial irregularity and localized edema had resolved; however, epithelial ingrowth was noted from 7 to 10 o'clock. Slit lamp photographs were taken.

At the 1-month visit, there was minimal progression of the epithelial ingrowth and the UCVA remained 20/20- 2. However, a stromal melt was noted in the area of the ingrowth. Corneal topographies were performed and he was scheduled for removal of the epithelial ingrowth.

On postoperative day 1, he had a UCVA of 20/30+2 and some rough epithelium inferiorly. He was given Ocuflox qid and chloramphenicol every 2 hours. Over the next few days he developed some mild localized stromal edema and was treated with tobramycin/dexamethasone and tapered off the Ocuflox and chloramphenicol.

By the 1-week examination there was some flap thinning with stromal loss from 8 to 9 o'clock and a small nest of epithelial cells at 7 o'clock. This was followed for 3 months. At this time, his UCVA was 20/15- 1 and the epithelial ingrowth remained unchanged. Slit lamp photographs were taken. We have continued to follow this patient every 2 to 3 months and have noticed no further changes.

The accompanying photographs and corneal map demonstrate the appearance and effect of the epithelial ingrowth and the stromal melt at varoius stages. This case illustrates that while a small nest of epithelial ingrowth can remain stable and without consequence, that a significant amount of ingrowth can cause a stromal melt and any should be removed promptly. Furthermore, with appropriate treatment, the flap can be stabilized and the vision excellent.

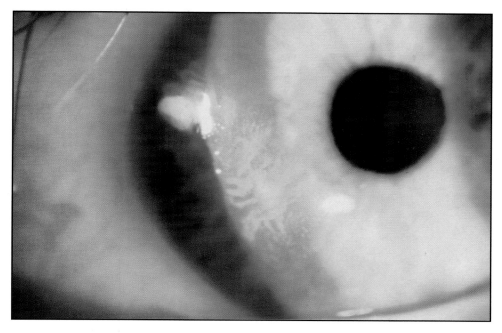

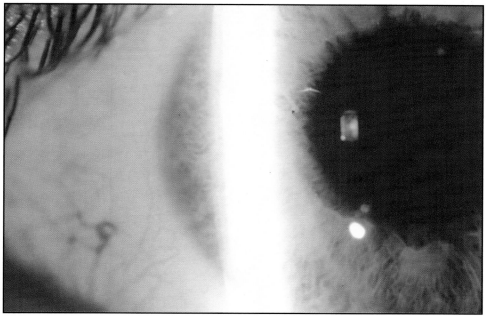

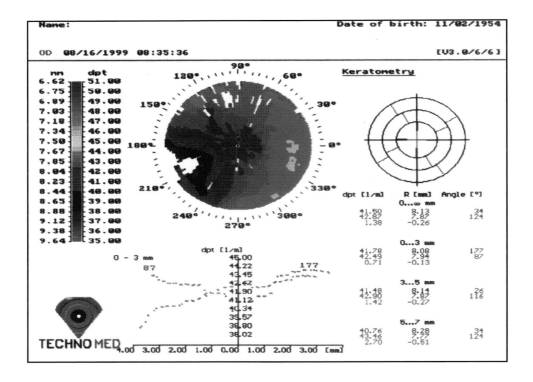

PATIENT EXAMPLE 17

Epithelial Basement Membrane Hypertrophy

This 39-year-old male underwent primary LASIK for myopic astigmatism OU. He was in good medical health, took no medications, and had no known drug allergies. Prior to surgery, the manifest refraction was -6.75 -2.75 x 5 corrected to 20/15 vision OD and -6.75 -3.00 x 169 corrected to 20/15 vision OS. During the LASIK procedure there was a small area of loose epithelium at 6 o'clock OD, so a contact lens was placed at the time of surgery. The postoperative course was unremarkable in the left eye. The epithelial looseness recovered quickly, but there were small microstriae in both eyes. The striae were not affecting visual acuity. An enhancement was performed 2 months postoperatively for plano -1.75 x 73 OD and 3 months postoperatively for -1.50 -0.50 x 59 OS.

The right eye recovered unremarkably and achieved an UCVA of 20/15. Mild stromal edema and small microstriae were noted postoperatively in the left eye 1 day after enhancement, but the UCVA was 20/15⁻² at this time. At the 1-month follow-up exam, there were a few more microstriae noted in the left eye, but the UCVA remained 20/15⁻¹. By the 3-month follow-up exam, there were microstriae and granular subepithelial irregularities centrally and the UCVA had decreased to 20/25⁻¹. By the fifth postoperative month, UCVA had decreased to 20/50 with a manifest refraction of -1.25 -0.75 x 80 corrected to 20/20⁻²—but with blurring and doubling. Slit lamp examination revealed central microstriae and nests of subepithelial basement membrane reduplication. Slit lamp photographs were taken, as well as corneal maps. A transepithelial PTK was scheduled to smooth the basement membrane and microstriae and to treat the residual myopia and astigmatism at the same time.

He recovered from the PTK unremarkably, and at the 1-week postoperative visit he had an UCVA of 20/15⁻¹ with a manifest refraction of +0.75 -0.25 x 177 with 20/15 OS. The basement membrane reduplication had resolved, and there were no microstriae. At the 2-month follow-up examination, his UCVA was 20/20⁻¹ and manifest refraction was +0.25 -0.50 x 130 to 20/20⁺². There was a 1.0 mm area of basement membrane irregularity outside the visual axis.

The accompanying photographs and corneal maps demonstrate the appearance and effect of the basement membrane reduplication at the fifth month after LASIK. This case demonstrates that microstriae that may be visually insignificant in themselves may lead to enough surface irregularity to develop basement membrane reduplication with a subsequent decrease in vision. This situation is best treated with a transepithelial PTK to remove the basement membrane reduplication and flatten the microstriae. Note that the PTK overtreatment had the effect of treating the residual myopia and astigmatism without performing a separate refractive PRK. Caution should be taken when performing a PTK on a patient with a plano refraction not to induce significant postoperative hyperopia.

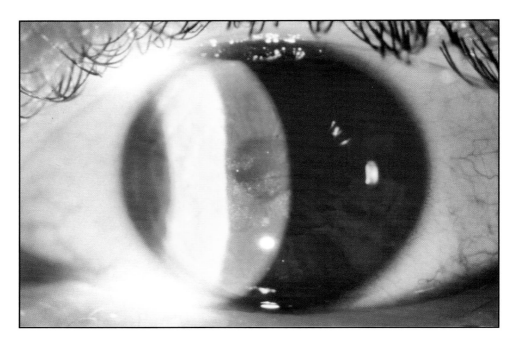

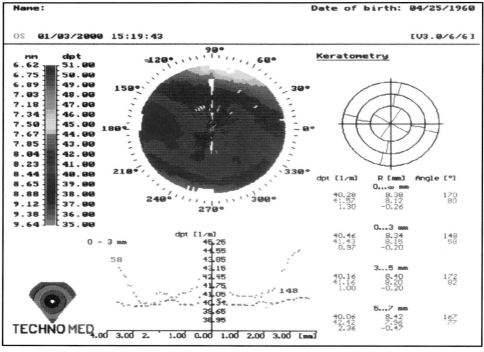

PATIENT EXAMPLE 18

Interface Haze

This patient was a 45-year-old man who had never worn contact lenses. His general health was good, and he never took medications. His uncorrected vision was 20/100 OD and 20/160 OS. Cycloplegic refraction showed +7.50 sphere with a vision of 20/30[-3] OD and +7.75 -0.75 x 55 with a best correction of 20/40 OS. Pachymetry was 0.479 OD and 0.482 OS. Manual keratometry was 40.87 @ 162 x 41.62 @ 72 OD and 40.75 @ 30 x 41.50 @ 120 OS. Corneal diameters were 11.75 OU. There was trace nuclear sclerosis OU. Reduced BCVA was felt to be due to deprivation amblyopia OU.

LASIK was performed OS; and at 4 days postoperative, VASC OS was 20/40[-1]. Slit lamp exam revealed trace crystal-like haze at the flap interface. LASIK was performed OD without complications. At 3 days postoperative, VASC was 20/40[-2], and slit lamp revealed trace refractile debris at the temporal margin and crystal-like haze centrally OD. At 5 months postoperative, VASC was 20/70[-2] OD and 20/50-1 OS, and cycloplegic refraction revealed +3.75 -1.25 x 150 OD and +1.75 -1.00 x 9 OS with a best corrected of 20/25[-2] OD and 20/30[-1] OS. Trace anterior stromal reticular haze was noted in a patchy pattern 3.0 mm in diameter centrally OD, and a similar pattern was noted OS.

At 2 months post-enhancement, VASC was 20/50[-1] OD and 20/40[-1] OS with a manifest refraction of +1.75 -0.75 x 35 OD corrected to 20/30[-2] and +1.25 sphere OS best corrected to +1.25 sphere OD and 20/40 OS. There was fine fibrosis of the flap incision OU and trace diffuse haze at the interface OU. The patient was happy with his vision at that time.

The accompanying maps demonstrate the preoperative and postoperative appearances in this case of hyperopic correction. The accompanying photograph shows the speckled-type haze that can be seen with some hyperopic corrections. This has been able to be reduced using a smoothing fluid after a hyperopic correction or an enhancement if we get that type of haze. Using smoothing fluid does seem to eliminate the occurrence of this haze, so it implies that it is due to an irregular surface from hyperopic ablations (which predisposes to this type of haze).

(Text and figures reprinted with permission from Gimbel HV, Anderson Penno EE. *LASIK Complications: Prevention and Management.* Thorofare, NJ: SLACK Incorporated, 1999.)

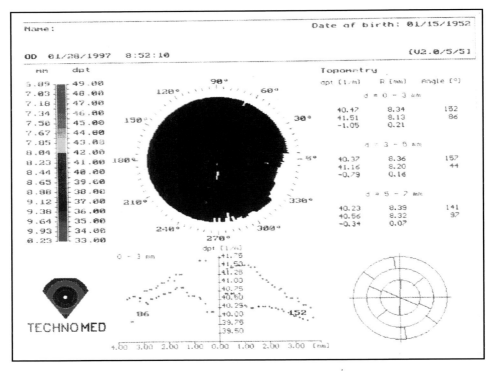

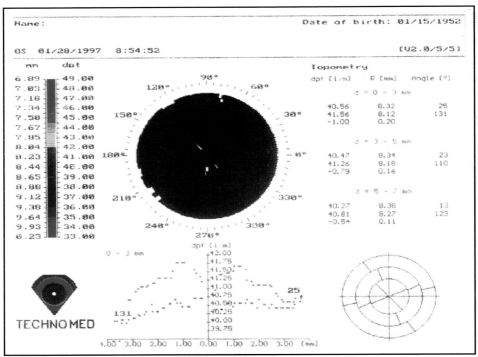

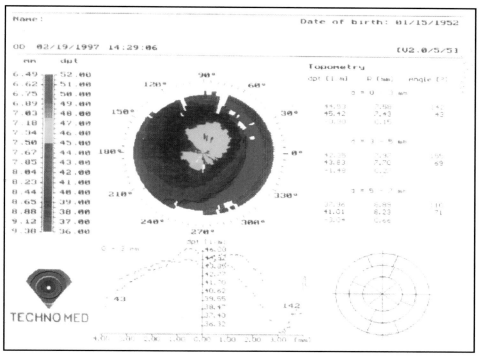

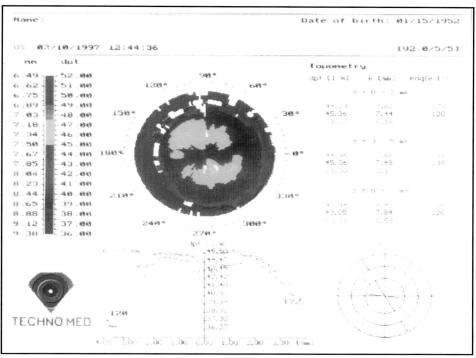

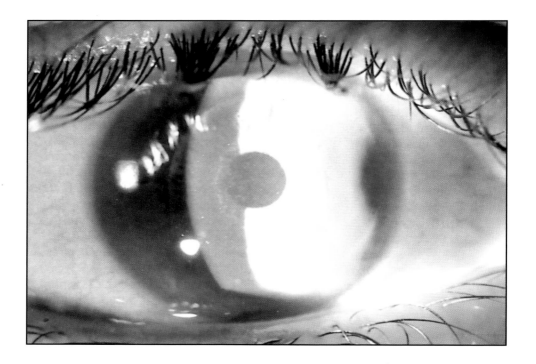

Diffuse Lamellar Keratitis

This patient was a 42-year-old female who occasionally wore contact lenses. She was in good medical health, took no medications, and was allergic to sulfa drugs. Her manifest refraction was -3.75 -0.25 x 55 with 20/20 vision OD and -2.50 -0.75 x 88 with 20/20 vision OS. Her cycloplegic refraction was -3.75 sphere OD and -2.25 -1.25 x 88 OS. Pachymetry was 0.522 μ OD and 0.505 μ OS. Slit lamp biomicroscopy and fundus examination were unremarkable.

Primary LASIK was performed OU with the left eye first and then the right eye second. The same blade was used for both eyes. During the LASIK procedure there was a small area of loose epithelium at 6 o'clock OS so a contact lens was placed in the left eye at the time of surgery. On the third postoperative day, her UCVA was 20/40⁺² pinhole to 20/20⁻² OD and 20/160 pinhole to 20/50⁻¹ OS with the contact lens. The right eye had SPK to explain the level of vision and the interface was clear. The left eye had diffuse interface inflammation with its typical crystal-like appearance (stage 2). The conjunctiva was minimally injected, as would be expected with loose epithelium. The epithelium was in place with no frank defect. There was no anterior chamber reaction and no pain. Slit lamp photography was performed.

The contact lens was removed and the patient was started on prednisolone acetate every hour and polymixin B sulfate six times a day in the left eye. The patient was followed closely and improved gradually. On postoperative day 7 she had UCVA of 20/30⁻¹ OS with a manifest refraction of -1.00 -4.00 x 80, 20/30⁻². Her examination revealed +2 to +3 central interface granularity measuring 4.5 x 3.0 mm. The medication was continued at the same frequency. The inflammation continued to decrease and the UCVA continued to improve over the next 3 weeks and the medication was slowly tapered. At the 1-month follow-up examination, her UCVA OS was 20/20⁻² with a manifest refraction of plano -0.50 x 180 20/20. She was on qid prednisolone acetate and polymixin B sulfate at this time. The polymixin B sulfate was discontinued and the prednisolone acetate was tapered one drop per week. She returned for her 3-month follow-up examination and the UCVA was 20/20⁻¹ with a manifest refraction of -0.25 -0.50 x 155 corrected to 20/15⁻². The interface inflammation had completely resolved. Slit lamp photographs were taken.

The accompanying photographs demonstrate the appearance of the interface inflammation and its resolution over time. This case demonstrates that with prompt care and treatment, there is the potential for complete recovery from significant interface inflammation.

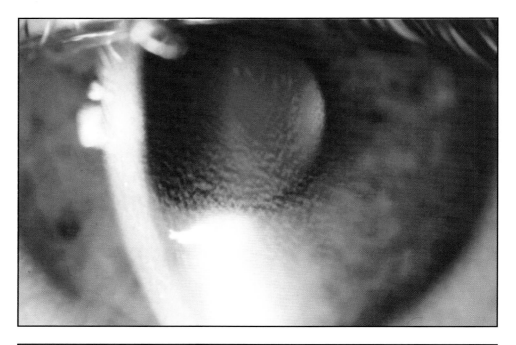

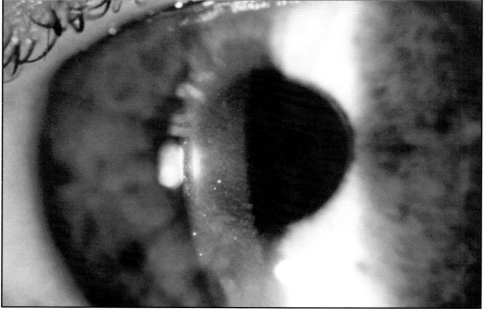

PATIENT EXAMPLE 20

Diffuse Lamellar Keratitis

This 48-year-old female underwent primary LASIK for myopic astigmatism OU. She was in good medical health, took no medications, and had no known drug allergies. Her manifest refraction on assessment was -5.75 -3.25 x 30 corrected to 20/20 [-3] OD and -5.00 -1.25 x 156 corrected to 20/20 [-3] vision OS. The postoperative course was unremarkable, but she remained undercorrected. A bilateral enhancement was performed 4 months postoperatively for -2.50 -1.75 x 15 OD and -2.00 -0.25 x 15 OS. Postoperatively, she had a UCVA and manifest refraction of 20/40 OD with -0.50 -2.25 x 22 corrected to 20/30 [+2] OD and a UCVA of 20/30 OS with -0.50 -0.50 x 135 corrected to 20/20 [-1] OS. The topographic map showed slight nasal decentration and a small, steep band of regular astigmatism centrally, which might account for the loss of BCVA. The patient was pleased with the results in the left eye but desired enhancement in the right eye. Calculated postoperative pachymetry of the residual bed OD was >250 microns, so a second enhancement was performed OD. The enhancement was uneventful.

On postoperative day 1, her UCVA was 20/40 [-1] pinholed to 20/25 OD. The right eye had mild interface inflammation circumferentially. There was no anterior chamber reaction and no pain. Prednisolone acetate and Ocuflox was started qid. Over the next 2 days, the inflammation increased slightly and the UCVA decreased to 20/70 [-1] pinholed to 20/20 [-1]. Polymixin B sulfate eye drops were added qid. Slit lamp photography was performed. On the sixth postoperative day, the UCVA was 20/50 with a manifest refraction of +1.00 -1.00 x 82 corrected to 20/30 [-2]. The patient had a mild epitheliopathy and the inflammation was unchanged so the prednisolone acetate was increased to every hour, and corneal topography was performed. Over the course of the next 3 months, the inflammation resolved and the medications were slowly tapered. However, her UCVA OD remained 20/40 and a manifest refraction of -0.50 -0.75 x 90 corrected to 20/25 [-1]. There is some mild peripheral epithelial ingrowth and surface irregularity, which may account for the loss of one-half a line of BCVA.

The accompanying photograph and corneal maps demonstrate the appearance and effect of the interface inflammation on the sixth postoperative day. This case demonstrates the potential refractive sequelle of interface inflammation and also illustrates that DLK may be encountered after enhancement procedures in which a microkeratome was not used.

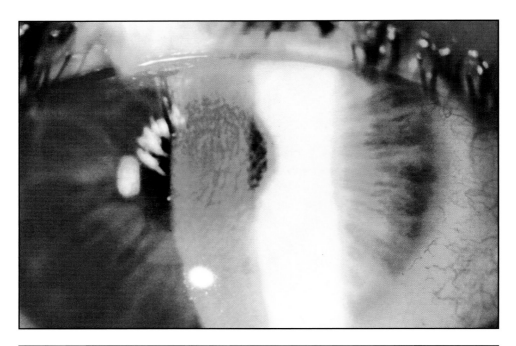

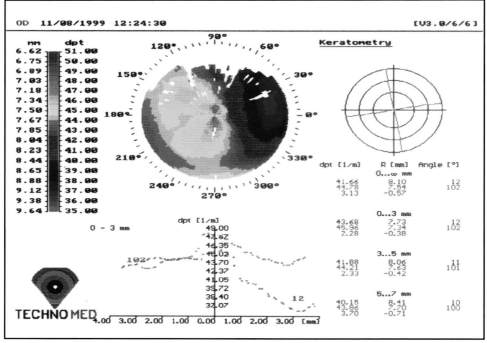

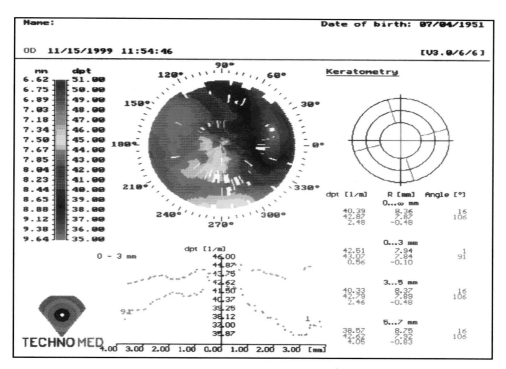

Name: Date of birth: 07/04/1951

OD   11/15/1999 11:54:46   [V3.0/6/6]

Keratometry

	mm	dpt
	6.62	51.00
	6.75	50.00
	6.89	49.00
	7.03	48.00
	7.18	47.00
	7.34	46.00
	7.50	45.00
	7.67	44.00
	7.85	43.00
	8.04	42.00
	8.23	41.00
	8.44	40.00
	8.65	39.00
	8.88	38.00
	9.12	37.00
	9.38	36.00
	9.64	35.00

	dpt [1/m]	R [mm]	Angle [°]
0...∞ mm	40.39	8.36	16
	42.87	7.87	106
	2.48	-0.48	
0...3 mm	42.51	7.94	1
	43.07	7.84	91
	0.56	-0.10	
3...5 mm	40.33	8.37	16
	42.79	7.89	106
	2.46	-0.48	
5...7 mm	38.57	8.75	16
	42.62	7.92	106
	4.06	-0.83	

TECHNO MED

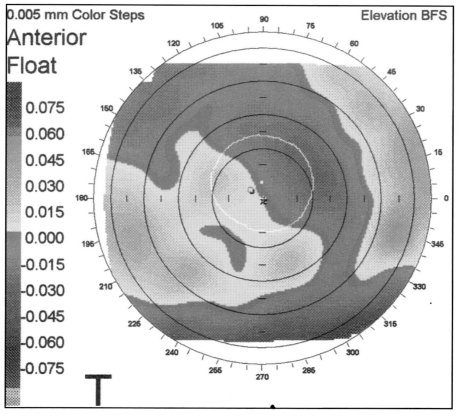

0.005 mm Color Steps   Elevation BFS

Anterior Float

0.075	
0.060	
0.045	
0.030	
0.015	
0.000	
-0.015	
-0.030	
-0.045	
-0.060	
-0.075	

T

Lamellar Keratitis Following Corneal Abrasion

This 38-year-old woman underwent uncomplicated bilateral LASIK for a refractive error of -4.25 -1.75 x 180 OD and -3.50 -1.75 x 162 OS. Preoperative BCVA was 20/20³ OU. Postocular and medical histories were negative and the preoperative examination was unremarkable. One day postoperatively, a 1.5 mm epithelial defect was noted along the nasal edge of the flap with a surrounding area of loose epithelium. The interface was clear. The patient was maintained on topical antibiotics and steroids. By postoperative day 3, UCVA was 20/25⁺³ OD and 20/25 OS and a small fusion line remained. At that visit, mild interface inflammation was noted underlying the fusion line and the patient was maintained on drops. By 1 week, the inflammation was resolving. At that visit, a manifest refraction was plano -1.00 x 17 OS with BCVA of 20/20.

The patient was seen 1 month postoperatively with a recurrent erosion at the nasal edge of the flap. No inflammation was noted. A combined steroid and antibiotic ointment was used until the defect healed. A small area of epithelial ingrowth was noted at the nasal flap edge.

At 6 months postoperatively, the patient presented with a 2-day history of a sore, irritated eye OS and photophobia. UCVA was 20/20⁻² OD and 20/50 OS. A fusion line was noted near the nasal edge of the flap with underlying interface inflammation. The patient was maintained on a combination steroid and antibiotic ointment. The epithelial ingrowth remained unchanged and the inflammation resolved within 1 week. At last follow-up 7 months postoperatively, UCVA was 20/20⁺² OD (OD dominant) and 20/25 OS with a manifest refraction of -0.50 -0.25 @ 151 OS. The cornea was quiet and epithelial ingrowth was unchanged.

This case demonstrates that interface inflammation can result from epithelial disruption and will resolve as the epithelium heals. The timing of interface inflammation following the primary LASIK and following the recurrent erosion at 6 months postoperatively was 2 to 3 days after the epithelial injury. In this case, the inflammation was localized to the area under the epithelial defect and should resolve with standard treatment.

Lamellar keratitis is discussed in Chapter 6. These cases should be followed closely to rule out the rare possibility of infectious keratitis. The case also demonstrates the increased risk of epithelial ingrowth in primary LASIK cases in which epithelial disruption occurs. In this case, a small area has been followed and no change was noted.

PATIENT EXAMPLE 22

Lamellar Keratitis Following Contact Lens Use

This 56-year-old woman presented 23 months after primary LASIK with a complaint of blurred vision OD. Manifest refraction revealed +1.25 -0.50 x 105 OD and plano OS. UCVA was 20/50 OD and 20/25⁻¹ OS (preoperative BCVA was 20/30 OU). Mild SPK was noted on slit lamp examination OU. A contact lens was recommended OD, and a slit lamp exam indicated a good fit of the contact lens.

The patient returned 4 days later complaining of irritation OD related to contact lens use. Slight staining was noted inferotemporally without an epithelial defect. Underlying interface inflammation was noted. Topical steroids and discontinuation of contact lens wear was recommended. One week later, UCVA was 20/40 OD and the interface inflammation had resolved. Mild SPK remained OD. Steroids were tapered and the interface remained quiet.

This case demonstrates that interface inflammation may result from irritation of the corneal surface (due to contact lens in this case). With discontinuation of the contact lens and appropriate treatment with topical antibiotics and steroids, the interface inflammation resolved.

PATIENT EXAMPLE 23

Severe Dry Eye

This 44-year-old female underwent primary LASIK for high myopic astigmatism OU. She was in good medical health, took iron pills only, and was allergic to sulfa drugs. Her manifest refraction on assessment was -8.75 -0.50 x 75 corrected to 20/20- 3 OD and -9.75 sphere corrected to 20/20-2 vision OS. Preoperatively she had no complaint of dry eyes but did have trace superficial punctate keratopathy inferiorly OU. Surgery OU was unremarkable.

On postoperative day 1 she had a UCVA of 20/40 OD and 20/50- 2 OS. Examination revealed trace SPK OD and moderate confluent SPK OS. Frequent artificial tears were advised. At the 1 week examination, she had complaints of dryness and her UCVA was now 20/40- 1 OD and 20/70- 1 OS. Examination showed 3+ SPK inferiorly OD and 4+ scattered SPK OS. Silicone punctal plugs were inserted in both inferior puncta and preservative-free artificial tears were recommended. Her UCVA improved over the next 3 months to 20/25+2 OD and 20/25- 3 OS, however the SPK were still present inferiorly OU. Silicone punctal plugs were inserted in both superior puncta at this visit. One month later, she returned with a feeling of fullness in the eyes related to the superior plugs; therefore, they were removed at this time. At the fifth postoperative month visit, rimexolone was added qid OU for persistent irritation. This was tapered over the next month to bid. On the 7 month postoperative examination, the UCVA was 20/50 OD and 20/60 OS. Blepharitis was noted, and the patient was started on lid scrubs and tobramycin/dexamethasone ointment qhs. At the 8th month visit, she was started on oral tetracycline 250 mg q.i.d. and the rimexolone was discontinued. She was last seen at her 11-month postoperative visit. UCVA was 20/20- 3 OD with a manifest refraction of plano -0.75 x 104 corrected to 20/20. UCVA OS was 20/25- 3 with a manifest refraction of plano -0.50 x 18 corrected to 20/25. She reported an improvement in VA OU but was still complaining of dryness. Examination of the lids revealed trace debris on the lashes. There were trace corneal SPK inferiorly. Tetracycline was continued at the same dosage for one more month. She was instructed to return in 6 months for follow-up.

Patients with dry eyes preoperatively need to be counseled regarding the persistence and possible worsening of their dry eye condition. In severe cases, this may be persistent for long periods of time and may be associated with a compromise in the visual acuity. This is even more important in patients with collagen vascular diseases. Glasses act as a protective barrier in front of the eyes, and they prevent evaporation of tears by about 40%. Dry eyes may worsen in some cases secondary to loss of that barrier.

PATIENT EXAMPLE 24

Night Vision Disturbance Postoperatively

This patient had PRK elsewhere for a preoperative refractive error of -11.25 -0.75 x 3 OD. An optical zone of 6 mm with transition zone to 7.0 mm was used. In spite of preoperative pupil measurements of only 4 mm in bright light and 6 mm in dim light, the patient experienced significant night vision difficulties with marked glare and halos.

Two years later, he was seen for a preoperative assessment for LASIK OD. His manifest refraction was -11.25 -0.75 x 2, best corrected to 20/20 OD. In spite of a UCVA of 20/15[-1], this patient elected to cancel surgery OD after the risks of night vision difficulties that might follow LASIK OD were discussed.

This patient felt that he was functioning well with a contact lens in his uncorrected eye. In spite of a large discrepancy between the two eyes and in spite of excellent uncorrected acuity post-PRK OS, this patient felt handicapped by the night vision disturbances that had occurred following PRK.

This emphasizes the importance of a careful preoperative discussion, which should include a discussion of the possibility of night vision disturbances even in patients whose pupils are not overly large (6 mm in dim light in this patient). This is more likely to pose a problem in high corrections, where there is a greater change in corneal contour between the untreated peripheral cornea and the treatment zone, and where the optical zone size may be limited by the depth of the ablation (see Figure 7-8).

(Reprinted with permission from Gimbel HV, Anderson Penno EE. *LASIK Complications: Prevention and Management.* Thorofare, NJ: SLACK Incorporated, 1999.)

PATIENT EXAMPLE 25

Night Vision Problems/Decentration

This 30-year-old woman had a history of gas permeable contact lens wear for 16 years. No other ocular or medical problems were noted except the use of asthma medications, including an inhaler. Uncorrected vision was count fingers 2 meters OU. Manifest refraction was -1.25 1.25 @ 180 corrected to 20/20- 1 OD and -9.50 -1.75 @ 170 20/20- 2 OS. Specular microscopy and pachymetry were normal. Keratometry was 44.50 @ 180 x 46.25 @ 90 OD and 44.37 @ 180 x 46.12 @ 90 OS. Pupils were 3.50 mm in bright light and 4.5 mm in dim light OU. The slit lamp and fundus exams were within normal.

LASIK was done OU without stabilizing the eyes with a Thornton ring. Poor centration and stability were noted intraoperatively. At the 4-month follow-up, the patient complained of night vision problems with halo and glare. These symptoms were disabling to the point of not being able to drive. She was satisfied with daytime driving. Uncorrected vision was 20/50 OD and 20/20- 2 OS. Cycloplegic refraction was +1.50 -1.25 @ 177 with vision of 20/25+2 OD and +0.75 sphere with vision 20/20 OS. Slit lamp showed flaps in good position OU with slight haze centrally OU and a few slight striae centrally OD. The patient was scheduled for enhancement and given pilocarpine 0.25% for use at night.

This example points out the importance of stability and centration during the ablation. Some surgeons feel that a Thornton ring can be used in all cases to avoid the initial startle reaction that patients often have from the noise at the beginning of the ablation with the loud popping sound that accompanies the laser ablation. If a Thornton ring is used, care should be taken as discussed in the text to ensure that the pupil is well-centered and that the cornea is not inadvertently rotated by pressure from the Thornton ring. This is illustrated in Figure 5-21. In this patient, the slight decrease in BCVA OD may have been due to centrally located striae. The night vision difficulties with accompanying halo and glare are likely due to decentration. The accompanying maps show preoperative and postoperative corneal maps. Retreatment strategies are discussed in Chapter 7.

(Text and figures reprinted with permission from Gimbel HV, Anderson Penno EE. *LASIK Complications: Prevention and Management.* Thorofare, NJ: SLACK Incorporated, 1999.)

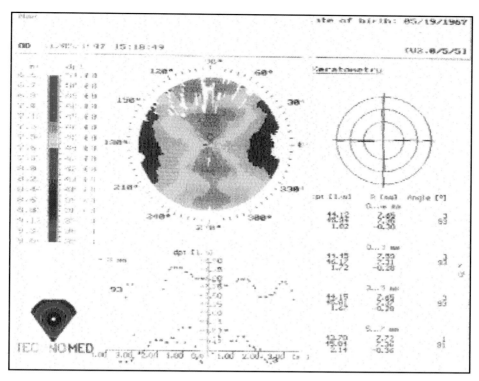

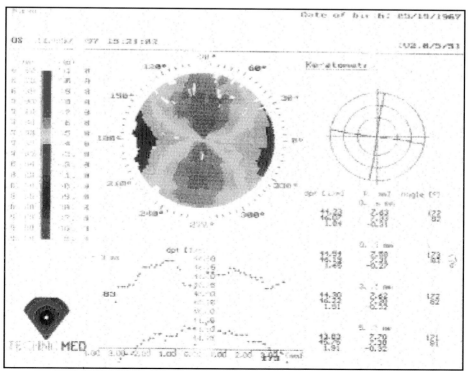

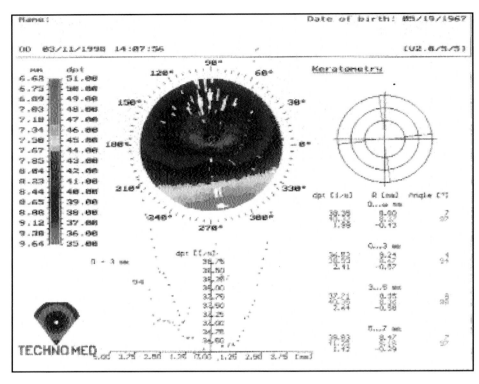

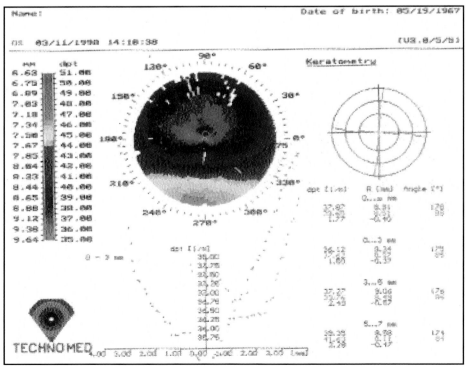

PATIENT EXAMPLE 26

Loose Epithelium on an Enhancement

This 46-year-old woman had a normal preoperative assessment and was scheduled for bilateral LASIK. Her manifest refraction was -1.50 -0.75 x 137 OD and -1.50 -0.50 x 166 OS with BCVA 20/20 OU. Keratometry readings were 44.50 @ 1.00 x 45.25 @ 91 OD and 44.75 @ 177 x 45.25 @ 87 OS. The anterior segment exam was unremarkable. LASIK OS was performed with significant loose epithelium encountered intraoperatively. The ablation was performed and a contact lens was placed. The surgeon and patient elected to perform PRK OS due to the risk of loose epithelium.

At 1 day postoperatively, UCVA was 20/60 OD and 20/125 OS. Significant sloughing of the loose epithelium had occurred in spite of the contact leaving >50% of the flap denuded. The patient complained of significantly more pain in the eye that had LASIK (OS). Epithelial remnants were removed and the contact lens was replaced. The patient was maintained on topic antibiotics until the epithelium healed.

By 3 months postoperatively, the UCVA was 20/20^{-2} OD and 20/60 OS with a manifest refraction of plano -0.75 x 171 OD and -0.25 -1.25 x 65 OS. BCVA was 20/15^{-1} OD and 20/20 OS. Enhancement was performed and again significant epithelial sloughing occurred, leaving a central 4 mm x 2.5 mm defect and a UCVA of 20/300 on postoperative day 1. The patient was maintained on topical antibiotics and a bandage contact lens was used until the defect healed. At 1 month post-enhancement OS (4 months postoperatively PRK OD), UCVA was 20/20 -0.25 x 170 OD and plano -0.80 x 80 OS. BCVA remained 10/10 OU.

This patient illustrates that the benefits of LASIK are lost (as compared to PRK) if significant epithelial disruption occurs. Every effort should be made to prevent epithelial disturbance as outlined in Table 5-14. Some surgeons test for loose epithelium on assessment by placing gentle traction on the corneal surface after placing topical anesthetic at the slit lamp. If loose epithelium is encountered on the first eye, there is an increased risk of epithelium on the second eye. Therefore, as was done in this case, consideration should be given to switching to PRK in the second eye if appropriate.

While large areas of epithelium do typically generally result from enhancements, if a significant epithelial problem occurred on the primary treatment, the patient should be advised that healing may be delayed following enhancement if epithelial disruption occurs again. This patient was much happier overall with her PRK experience as compared to her difficult postoperative course with her LASIK eye. At her last follow-up, she was pleased with her overall vision.

Thin Flap: Unable to Lift Flap on Enhancement

This was a 24-year-old woman who had no previous medical problems with a history of esotropia with amblyopia OD. The only medication she was taking was birth control pills. Her UCVA was 20/30⁻³ OD and 20/30 OS. The cycloplegic refraction was +3.00 -0.25 x 170 correctable to 20/20 OD and +2.00 -0.50 x 170 correctable to 20/20 OS. Corneal diameters were 12.50 mm OU. Manual keratometry was 41.75 @ 8 x 43.00 @ 98 OD and 41.75 @ 175 x 42.75 @ 85 OS. Slit lamp and fundus exams were normal.

LASIK was performed OU without complications. At 1 month postoperatively, VASC OD was 20/20⁻³ with a manifest refraction of +0.25 -0.25 x 19 and VASC was 20/30⁻² OS with a manifest of 0.25 -1.00 x 135 with vision of 20/20⁻². There was fine fibrosis at the incision site and a horizontal band of diffuse haze at the superior pupillary margin OS. There was trace diffuse haze noted OU.

At 3.5 months postoperatively, VASC OD was 20/25⁺² and VA OS was 20/30⁻². The cycloplegic refraction was +0.25 -1.00 x 168 with a cycloplegic vision of 20/20 OS. It was noted at that time that there were no wrinkles or folds in the flap, but there was an area of the flap at the superior edge OS that appeared thin.

LASIK enhancement was attempted OS; however, there was no laser treatment performed because the surgeon was unable to lift the flap completely. The flap was replaced to its original position and irrigated with BSS. One month after the enhancement attempt, VASC OS was 20/25⁻³ and the manifest refraction was plano -1.00 x 170 best corrected to 20/20⁻¹. It was decided that an attempt to recut the flap would be made in 2 months.

This is a fairly uncommon case in which an adherent flap was encountered and enhancement by lifting the flap was not possible. It would seem that the hyperopic ablation left an irregular surface compared to myopic ablations and that excessive fibrosis occurred in the interface. In cases such as these, the flap should be allowed to heal and then plan to recut the flap for the enhancement.

(Reprinted with permission from Gimbel HV, Anderson Penno EE. *LASIK Complications: Prevention and Management*. Thorofare, NJ: SLACK Incorporated, 1999.)

PATIENT EXAMPLE 28

Adherent LASIK Flap Recut

This 27-year-old man had a history of patching OD when he was young and a history of his OS turning in. His UCVA was 20/25⁻³ OD and 20/50⁻² OS. The manifest refraction was +4.50 -1.25 x 180 with best-corrected vision of 20/20⁻² OD. The manifest refraction OS was +6.50 -1.75 x 20, with vision of 20/30⁻³. Cycloplegic refraction OD was +6.00 -1.75 x 172 with vision of 20/20, and cycloplegic refraction was +7.00 -1.75 x 16 with vision of 20/40 OS. Manual keratometry was 40.50 @ 162 x 43.00 @ 72 OD and 40.62 @ 14 x 42.75 @ 104 OS. Corneal diameters were 11.25 OU. The slit lamp and fundus exams were normal.

LASIK was performed without complications OU. At the 5-month follow-up visit, the patient's UCVA was 20/30⁻² OD and 20/30⁻³ OS. The patient noted shadows below the letters OD. The manifest refraction was -1.00 -2.00 x 177 with vision of 20/20 OD and +2.25 -1.75 x 30 with of 20/30⁻² OS. It was noted that there was mild haze OU along flap incision and hinges. Also, a ring of mild stromal haze was noted midperiphery OU with central clearing.

An enhancement was attempted OD, 6 months after the original surgery. The flap was noted to be adherent at the 5 to 6 mm zone and could not be lifted; therefore, laser ablation was not performed. The patient was advised to wait until the edges of the flap had resealed and corneal maps and refraction were stable. Approximately 7 weeks later, an enhancement was done on the right eye with a recut of the flap. At 4 days postoperative, LASIK enhancement uncorrected vision was 20/20 OD with a manifest refraction of +0.25 sphere. The flap was in good position. There was a fine microstriation at the flap hinge and mild fibrosis along the flap incision. Again, mild haze was found in a ring-shaped pattern OD. At 2 months postoperatively, the vision remained 20/20 without correction, and the patient was pleased.

This is an uncommon case in which the flap was unable to be lifted at the time of enhancement and was replaced and allowed to heal. A recut was to be made for the subsequent enhancement, as was performed in this case. This case also demonstrated the mild annular haze that can be seen following hyperopic corrections (as demonstrated in Patient Example 18).

(Reprinted with permission from Gimbel HV, Anderson Penno EE. *LASIK Complications: Prevention and Management.* Thorofare, NJ: SLACK Incorporated, 1999.)

PATIENT EXAMPLE 29

RK/LASIK/PTK

This 39-year-old woman was 10 years postoperative RK OD, and 9 years postoperative RK OS. She stated that she was having some difficulty at night. Her vision fluctuated, and she was concerned with halos. Her vision without correction was 20/20 OD and 20/30- 2 OS. A cycloplegic refraction revealed +0.25 -0.25 x 134 best corrected to 20/15- 1 OD and +2.25 -0.75 x 58 best corrected to 20/20 OS. Manual keratometry showed 41.75 @ 144 x 42.37 @ 54 and 39.37 @ 24 x 40.50 @ 114 OS with slightly distorted mires OU. Her IOPs were normal. There was fine fibrosis of the incisions OD with no gaping, and incisions were clean with no gaping OS. The slit lamp and fundus exams were within normal.

LASIK was performed without complication OS; and at 3 days postoperatively, the patient complained of extreme blurriness in the left eye. Uncorrected vision was 20/250. The flap had shifted with striations running obliquely and centrally through the flap. The patient was brought back to the operating room, the flap was lifted, and the stromal side of the flap and stromal bed were wiped with a Paton spatula to smooth and remove epithelial tags. The corneal flap was moistened and replaced to the original position. Fluid was then dried from the edges.

One month postoperatively, her vision without correction was 20/50 OS, and her manifest refraction was -0.25 -1.00 x 10 (correctable to 20/20- 3 OS). There was fine fibrosis of the radial and flap incisions. The flap was in good position with a clean interface. It was felt that there was a whitish opacity, possibly an epithelial nest, in the RK incision at 1 o'clock at the edge of the flap.

This patient returned at the 2-month postoperative visit with uncorrected vision of 20/30 OS. Her manifest refraction was 0.00 -0.75 x 8 with best corrected of 20/20- 1 OS. At the 5-month visit, she complained of monocular diplopia OS, especially in the top half of letters. Her vision without correction was 20/25- 2, and manifest refraction was 0.00 -1.00 x 178 best corrected to 20/20 OS. It was felt that there was some irregular astigmatism and filamentary keratitis as well. The corneal map showed some inferior flattening.

At the 6.5-month postoperative LASIK visit, her uncorrected vision was 20/25- 2 and a cycloplegic refraction revealed 0.00 -0.50 x 175 with a best-corrected vision of 20/20+2. PTK was performed, and it showed central epithelial breakthrough. Smoothing was done with sodium hyaluronate. At the 2-month postoperative visit, the patient stated that vision fluctuated. Her vision without correction was 20/40- 1, and the manifest refraction was +1.00 -1.50 x 56 with a best-corrected vision of 20/20- 3. There was mild diffuse SPK, and the radial incisions were clear. The patient was noted to have lagophthalmos OS and was instructed to use ointment at bedtime, as well as liberal artificial tears during the day.

This patient's shifted flap is demonstrated in Figure 8-3. This photograph nicely demonstrates the misalignment of the incisions in the flap and bed, which can be a sensitive indicator of flap position. In this case, PTK was also attempted for treatment of irregular astigmatism. The advantages and disadvantages of LASIK or PRK after RK are outlined in Tables 8-1a and b. In this case, a combined approach was taken, whereby LASIK was performed for correction of hyperopia followed by PTK for attempted correction of irregular astigmatism.

LASIK after RK can pose a risk for epithelial ingrowth and ectasia. This is of particular concern if there are epithelial gaping RK incisions with epithelial plugs. In patients who are noted to have epithelial plugs preoperatively, consideration should be given to performing PRK, but the decision whether to perform PRK versus LASIK will be dependent on the presence or absence of surface irregularities, as well as the magnitude of the overall correction.

(Reprinted with permission from Gimbel HV, Anderson Penno EE. *LASIK Complications: Prevention and Management.* Thorofare, NJ: SLACK Incorporated, 1999.)

PATIENT EXAMPLE 30

LASIK over Epikeratophakia

This 31-year-old woman had a history of epikeratophakia OD, and a graft replacement in 1987. The patient states that after about 2 years, vision decreased enough to need correction. She wore soft lenses OU. Her uncorrected vision was 20/400 OD. The manifest refraction was -3.25 -3.00 x 20 corrected to 20/20⁻ ¹ OD and -8.25 -0.75 at 145 correctable to 20/20 OS. Manual keratometry was 39.12 @ 35 x 43.50 @ 125 OD and 43.00 @ 164 x 43.75 @ 74 OS. Slit lamp revealed trace haze around the tucking of the epi button, which was 9 mm in diameter with an exposed area of 6.5 mm in diameter OD. The lenticule appeared to be about 200 μm thick from the measurements. Slit lamp exam of the lens revealed cortical spoking at 5 and 6 o'clock OD and peripheral cortical spoking at 4 o'clock OS. It was felt that there may be less haze potential with LASIK, and the patient elected to proceed. Surgery was uneventful. No separation of tissue occurred. An ablation of -1.46 -3.00 x 25 was performed.

At 1 day postoperative, uncorrected vision OD was 20/20 with a manifest refraction of +6.25 -1.00 x 135. Vision was 20/20 OD. The refraction at 2 days postoperative was +4.50 -0.50 x 163, VASC remained 20/20. The patient stated that her near vision was somewhat difficult with small print.

LASIK was performed OS 3 months later for correction of -6.75 - 0.75 x 157; and at 1 day postoperative, VASC was 20/20⁻ ¹ with a manifest refraction of +2.00 -1.00 x 113. At 6 months postoperative LASIK over epikeratophakia OD and 3 months postoperative primary LASIK OS, VASC was 20/70⁻ ¹ OD and 20/25 OS. The manifest refraction was +4.00 -1.75 x 180 OD corrected to 20/20⁻ ¹ and 0.00 -0.50 x 135 OS corrected to 20/15⁻ ². There were no wrinkles or folds in the flap OU.

An enhancement was performed OD by lifting the flap 6 months after the original surgery. At 4 days after enhancement OD, VASC was 20/20⁻ ¹, manifest refraction was +1.75 -0.75 x 160 corrected to 20/20⁻ ¹. The patient was happy with her vision.

While the experience at our center includes only a few patients, the results indicate that LASIK after epikeratophakia is safe. This patient had an unexpected overcorrection that resulted in the decision to do a planned staged procedure that was performed successfully on a subsequent patient (see Patient Example 31). The accompanying maps demonstrate the preoperative state, 1 day after the primary procedure, preoperative enhancement corneal map, and the map at 4 days postoperative enhancement of the right eye. This case suggests that in addition to planning a staged procedure, a conservative approach should be taken with regard to laser ablation parameters when doing LASIK over previous epikeratophakia.

(Text and figures reprinted with permission from Gimbel HV, Anderson Penno EE. *LASIK Complications: Prevention and Management.* Thorofare, NJ: SLACK Incorporated, 1999.)

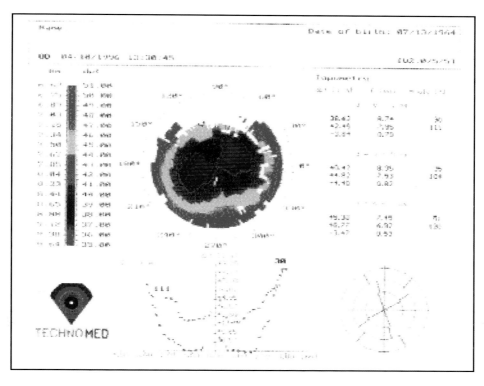

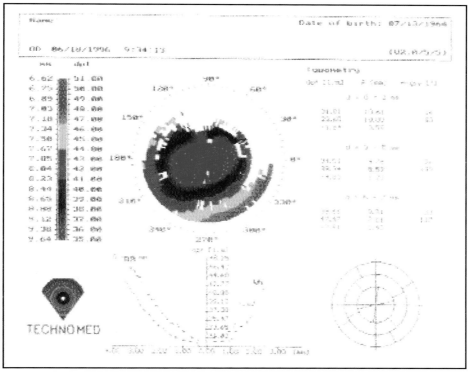

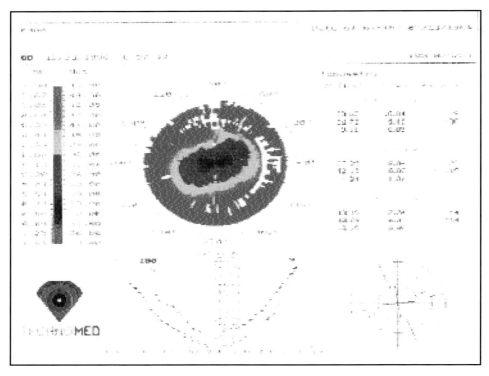

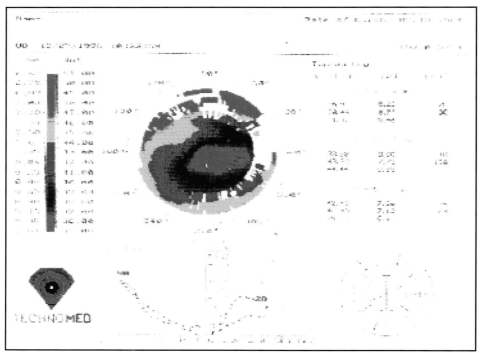

PATIENT EXAMPLE 31

LASIK over Epikeratophakia

This is a 57-year-old woman with a history of having had epikeratophakia OU (BKS, 6 mm shallow trephination and a 9 mm lenticule) approximately 10 years earlier. She was taking no medications and was in good general health. Her uncorrected vision was 20/160 OD and 20/40[-1] OS. Cycloplegic refraction revealed + 0.50 -7.00 x 42 OD best corrected to 20/25 OD and +3.25 -3.50 x 147 best corrected to 20/25[-2] OS. Pachymetry was 0.755 mm OD and 0.715 mm OS. Manual keratometry revealed 40.50 @ 45 x 42.75 @ 135 OD and 37.37 @ 35 x 34.25 @ 125 OS. Corneal diameters were 11.50 mm OU. The slit lamp exam revealed mild fibrosis at the periphery of the graft OU, with mild stromal granularity centrally OD. There was a running suture in place OS and 1+ nuclear sclerosis OU. The funduscopic exam was within normal.

Because of unexpected overcorrection that occurred in a previous patient, a staged LASIK procedure was planned. The first stage of the LASIK procedure was done OD with simply a cut being made with no laser ablation. At 3 days, VASC OD was 20/30[-3], and a manifest refraction revealed -0.25 sphere with a manifest vision of 20/30[-3]. The flap was noted to be in good position.

In this case, simply performing the LASIK cut over epikeratophakia resulted in a dramatic reduction of the preoperative astigmatism. To date, this patient has not required any laser ablation. The accompanying maps demonstrated the preoperative state and 3 day postoperative appearance of the corneal maps.

(Text and figures reprinted with permission from Gimbel HV, Anderson Penno EE. *LASIK Complications: Prevention and Management.* Thorofare, NJ: SLACK Incorporated, 1999.)

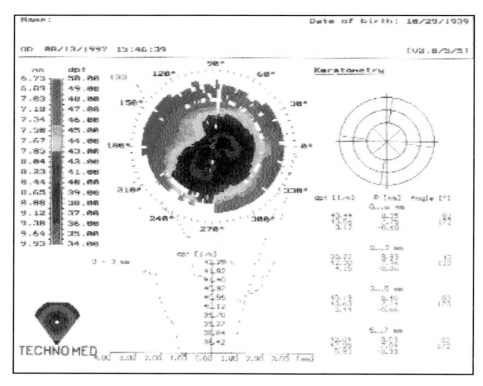

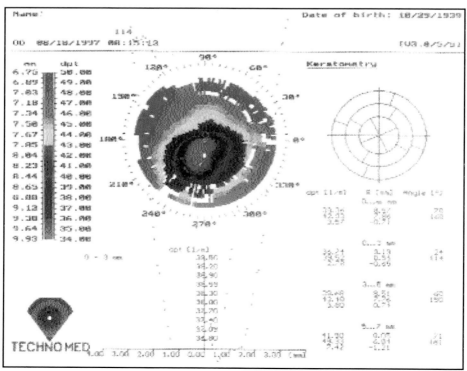

PATIENT EXAMPLE 32

LASIK over PKP

This 32-year-old man had PKP in 1986 OS and in 1981 for keratoconus OU. He had a history of wearing rigid gas permeable lenses 10 to 12 hours a day OU. His uncorrected vision was count fingers OU. His vision was 20/25⁻³ with a contact lens OD. A manifest refraction of -4.25 -6.75 x 160 gave a best-corrected vision of 20/60⁻² OS. The grafts were clear OU. Manual keratometries were 39.75 @ 167 x 49.37 @ 76 with distorted mires OS. Corneal diameter was 12.25 mm. The lens was noted to have trace nuclear sclerosis and trace cortical changes OS. Endothelial cell counts were 1400 OD and 550 OS. Pachymetry was within normal OU.

It was recommended that the patient undergo a two-stage LASIK approach OS. First, do the microkeratome cut only; and then a few days later, re-refract and then do the laser ablation. The patient had a Chiron ACS microkeratome cut as the first stage of LASIK OS using a 160 µm depth plate. The flap was very thin with the epithelium intact and a Bowman's buttonhole. At 3 days postoperative, the cornea OS was noted to have a patch of rough epithelium centrally, with SPK overlying. It was noted that the flap was very thin over a 2 to 2.5 mm zone, slightly off-center nasally where only the epithelium was in the flap; however, the epithelium was not broken.

One month after the LASIK cut OS, VASC was count fingers at 1.5 meters, and his vision with a contact OS was 20/20⁻². The manifest refraction was -5.00 -7.50 x 159 with a vision of 20/50⁻¹. There was noted to be fine fibrosis at the flap incision, an irregular rectangular faint perimeter haze about 2 mm wide corresponding to the edge of the buttonhole. Shortly after the first month visit, the flap was then successfully recut with the Hansatome using a 180 µ depth plate. Laser correction was also performed at this time. At 3 days postoperative, VASC was 20/200, with a manifest refraction +1.75 -5.75 x 174 and best corrected of 20/50⁻² OS. An enhancement was done for under-response at that time.

Four months after enhancement surgery, visual acuity was 20/40⁻¹ uncorrected OS with a manifest refraction of +2.00 -1.50 x 161 correctable to 20/40⁻² (with spectacles). A second enhancement was performed by lifting the flap; and 1 week postoperatively the uncorrected vision was 20/100 OS with a manifest refraction of -2.75 -1.75 x 85 correctable to 20/30⁻¹ (with spectacles). The over-response to plus cylinder correction required further enhancement.

The accompanying corneal maps demonstrate the appearance preoperatively, at the 1-month post-LASIK cut, and at 4 months after the first enhancement. There is persistent astigmatism throughout, although much improved. This patient's best spectacle-corrected visual acuity has improved from 20/60⁻² to 20/30⁻¹. The myopia following the final enhancement may be expected to diminish to some degree over time. This has been the experience with hyperopic corrections.

Steep grafts (particularly high cylinder corneas) are at a greater risk for button-holes and thin flaps. In addition, caution is advised with patients in whom the peripheral cornea is quite thin, such as can occur in keratoconus patients. If thinning is present in the peripheral cornea, consideration should be given to performing PRK.

This case demonstrates that LASIK with multiple enhancements can be safely performed after PKP; however, the graft's response to laser ablation may be variable.

(Text and figures reprinted with permission from Gimbel HV, Anderson Penno EE. *LASIK Complications: Prevention and Management.* Thorofare, NJ: SLACK Incorporated, 1999.)

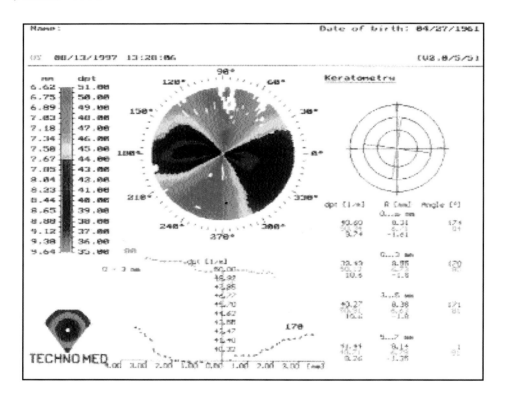

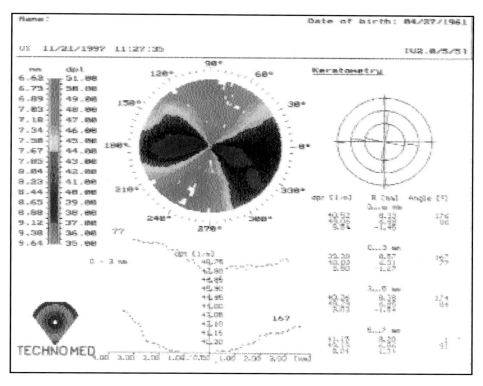

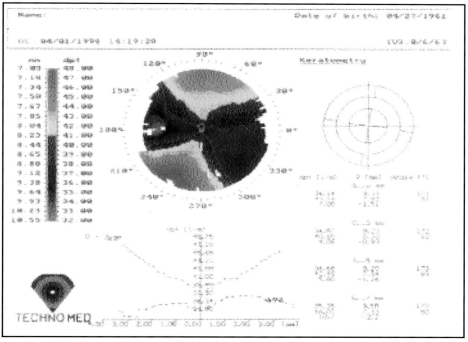

LASIK over PRK

This 41-year-old woman had a history of strabismus. Her general medical health was good, and she was taking no ocular or systemic medications. Her uncorrected vision was 20/400 OU. The manifest refraction was +7.75 sphere with a best-corrected vision of 20/30⁻³ OD and +7.75 -0.75 x 178 best corrected to 20/15⁻² OS. Manual keratometry was 42.25 @ 12 x 43.12 @ 102 OD and 42.62 @ 9 x 44.25 @ 99 OS. Her IOPs were normal. Slit lamp exam was within normal. The patient was left-eye dominant.

Hyperopic PRK was performed OD using a 5.5 mm optical zone and a 9.0 mm transition zone. The patient was maintained on topical steroids for 3 months following PRK. At 6 months postoperatively, the uncorrected vision OD was 20/50⁻¹. A cycloplegic refraction revealed +3.75 -1.00 x 150, best corrected to 20/30⁻³. The slit lamp revealed trace ring haze at the 4.5 to 5 mm zone.

LASIK was performed OS using the ACS 6 months later with a 5.5 optical zone and a transition zone of 9 mm without complications. The flap diameter was 8.75 mm and the hinge area was shielded during ablation. At 8 months postoperative PRK OD and 2.5 months post-hyperopic LASIK OS, uncorrected vision was 20/60⁻¹ with a manifest of +3.00 -1.25 x 163 and best corrected of 20/30⁻¹ OD, and uncorrected vision OS was 20/25 with a manifest of +1.25 -1.50 x 11 corrected to 20/20. The slit lamp exam revealed moderate ring-shaped haze with a reticular pattern greatest nasally, central clearing OD and moderate reticular haze centrally with moderate haze along the flap incision OS. In addition, one focal spot of stromal haze at 1 o'clock close to the flap edge was noted OS.

Hyperopic LASIK enhancement was performed OS. The focal haze, noted previously, appeared at the time of surgery to be an epithelial nest, and this area was debrided at the time of enhancement. A PRK enhancement was done on that date as well on the right eye. The patient was placed on topical steroids again for 3 months postoperatively. Three months after the enhancement in both eyes, the patient stated that the left eye seemed to fluctuate, particularly in the past 2 weeks. UCVA was 20/40⁻¹ OD and 20/20⁻³ OS. The cycloplegic refraction revealed +0.75 -0.50 x 1 OD corrected to 20/40 and +1.75 -1.00 x 4 corrected to 20/20 OS. The slit lamp revealed an arc of mild haze nasally OD and two areas of epithelial interface opacities at 12 o'clock and 1:30 with a ring of iron deposition as well OS.

Enhancement was performed OS, and in addition to retreating the residual hyperopia and astigmatism, the areas of presumed epithelial ingrowth were also cleared. At 8 months post-PRK enhancement OD and 5 months post-LASIK enhancement OS, the patient again complained of fluctuating vision OS. The UCVA was 20/70⁻² OD and 20/20⁻¹ OS. A cycloplegic refraction showed +6.00 -1.00 x 159 best corrected to 20/40⁺² OD and + 0.50 -0.75 x 148 best corrected to 20/20⁺³ OS. The slit lamp exam revealed a moderately dense ring of haze in the midperiphery OD, with moderately dense haze at the edge of the flap OS, with a small spot of haze in the midperiphery at 4:30. No epithelial ingrowth was noted OS.

Because of haze and regression, LASIK enhancement over PRK was performed in the right eye 11 months after the last PRK enhancement. Approximately 5 months after LASIK enhancement OD, UCVA was 20/60- OD and 20/25- OS. Manifest refraction was +2.00 +0.75 x 65 best corrected to 20/30- OD and -0.25 + 0.75 x 125 best corrected to 20/20+ OS. There was annular reticular stromal haze with central involvement OD and residual interface scarring in a ring pattern OS.

The accompanying photographs demonstrate the appearance of the right and left eyes following the primary procedures prior to any enhancements and the appearance at latest follow-up. The area of epithelial ingrowth at the 1 o'clock position in the left eye after the primary surgery is not clearly demonstrated in these photographs; however, one can appreciate the appearance of haze OU. This case reflects our early experience with hyperopic PRK and hyperopic LASIK. We no longer do hyperopic PRK for new cases because we have found, as is demonstrated in this case, that hyperopic patients tend to show haze and regression following PRK. As is demonstrated in this and previous cases (see Patient Example 18), there can be annular interface haze following hyperopic LASIK as well.

This example also demonstrates the risk for epithelial ingrowth that occurs when hyperopic corrections with a large transition zone are performed. In this case, a 5.5 mm optical zone with a transition zone of 9 mm was used, and this case was performed with the ACS, which creates a smaller flap than does the newer Hansatome. The larger flap and bed created by the Hansatome may be an advantage in performing hyperopic LASIK. The surgeon must be careful to avoid spillover of the laser ablation onto the edge of the stromal bed, particularly at the hinge area. If necessary, the hinge should be shielded with a sponge.

(Text and figures reprinted with permission from Gimbel HV, Anderson Penno EE. *LASIK Complications: Prevention and Management.* Thorofare, NJ: SLACK Incorporated, 1999.)

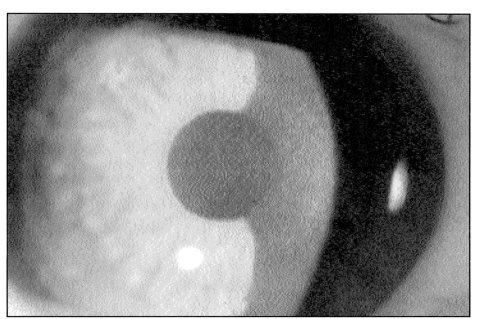

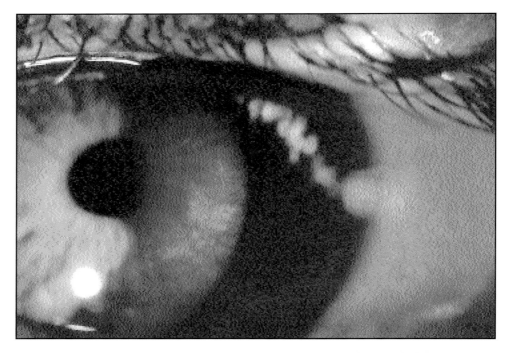

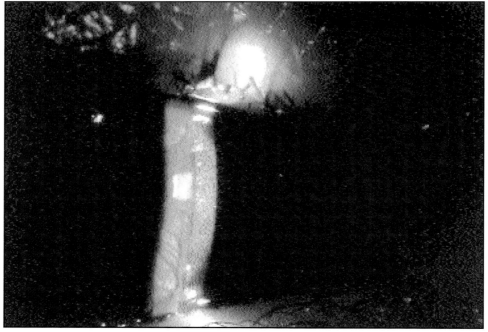

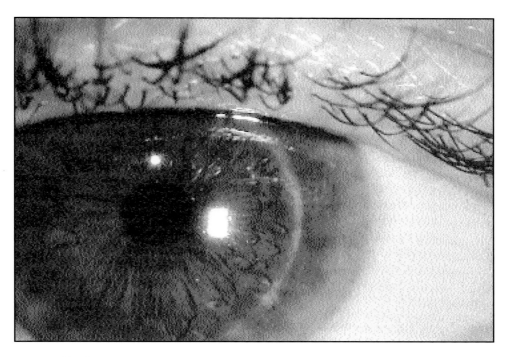

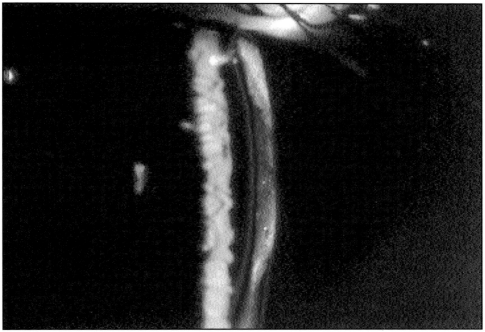

PATIENT EXAMPLE 34

PRK over LASIK

This 34-year-old woman had a history of hard contact lens use, no medical or ocular problems, took no medications, and was right-eye dominant. Uncorrected vision was count fingers at 1 meter OU. The manifest refraction was -13.50 -2.25 x 23, with manifest vision of 20/20⁻² OD and -15.25 -2.75 x 154 with manifest vision of 20/25⁻² OS. Manual keratometry readings were 44.12 @ 15 x 46.12 @ 105 OD and 44.37 @ 161 x 46.75 @ 71 OS. Pupil diameters were 5.0 mm in bright light and 7.00 mm in dim light. Slit lamp and funduscopic exams were within normal.

LASIK was performed using the ACS and the Nidek laser with a 5.5 mm optical zone with a transition zone to 7.0 mm OS. Intraoperatively, it was noted that there was slight central thinning of the flap. The laser ablation was performed. At 1 day postoperatively, some epithelial irregularities were noted. It was described as a pseudodendrite; and by 4 months postoperatively, it was noted that there was some superficial haze in a corresponding dendritic pattern. The patient was started on FML. Throughout the postoperative period, the refraction remained stable. The UCVA at the 6-month visit was 20/100, with a manifest refraction of -1.75 -1.25 x 152 correctable to 20/30⁻². It was felt that the decrease in vision was due to the fine haze centrally.

At 13 months postoperative LASIK OS, UCVA remained 20/100 with a manifest refraction of -2.00 -2.25 x 160 best corrected to 20/30⁻². Haze was still noted centrally. A PRK enhancement was decided upon and it was felt that laser ablation of the epithelium should be done due to the previous thin flap. Initially, a hyperopic PRK pattern of 5.5 mm optical zone and 7.0 mm transition zone was done in the epithelium. PTK with a 5.5 mm transition to 7 mm was done until breakthrough, which started peripherally. Myopic PRK was then done with parameters of -1.91 -2.25 x 160 at a zone from 5.5 to 7.0 mm to ablate the central epithelium. There was still no breakthrough centrally and, again, more peripheral breakthrough, so another diopter of myopic PRK 5.5 to 7.0 mm was used. Breakthrough was then quite uniform. Because of the previous peripheral breakthrough, near full correction PRK was used for refractive PRK.

At 3.5 months postoperative PRK enhancement, UCVA was 20/60⁻², the cycloplegic refraction was +7.25 -1.75 x 167, best corrected to 20/25⁺¹ OS. Central reticular haze began to develop; by 15 months, the UCVA was 20/125, and the manifest refraction was -2.75 -5.00 x 165 with vision of 20/40⁻². Moderate anterior stromal reticular haze was noted in a contiguous diffuse 3 mm circular pattern centrally. A PRK pattern was performed on the epithelium followed by PTK with a treatment zone of 5.0. The patient remained on FML tid; at the 3-month follow-up visit after the second enhancement, the VASC was 20/40⁻² with manifest refraction stabilizing at +0.50 -1.5 x 163 with a BCVA of 20/25⁻¹. There was still some mild haze in a 5 to 6 mm zone centrally. The patient was continued on FML topical drops three times a day.

In this case, the average keratometry readings do fall within the normal range, and one would not have suspected that this patient would have been at risk for a thin flap or buttonhole (although the average keratometry readings are at the higher end of normal). The surgeon elected to continue with the laser ablation at the primary surgery. This was early in our experience and we had not yet learned that with thin flaps, performing the ablation adds to the risk of haze and irregular astigmatism; repositioning the flap and recutting at a deeper plane a few months later for the refractive ablation reduces the risk of haze when a thin flap is obtained. Subsequently, because of the thin flap and haze, it was elected to proceed with PTK and PRK for correction of residual myopia.

As is demonstrated in this case, there is an increased risk of haze when proceeding with ablation after a thin flap is created, and the patient did develop reticular haze in a contiguous diffuse 3 mm pattern centrally. Superficial PTK may be useful for surface irregularities. However, in cases like this, we would advise recutting a deeper flap for definitive refractive correction in the presence of slight haze in Bowman's membrane as a result of flaps or buttonholes. To reduce the risk of haze, we advise repositioning the flap when a thin flap or buttonhole occurs in a primary LASIK procedure rather than proceeding with the laser ablation. In these cases, it is advisable to recut the flap at a later date.

(Text and figures reprinted with permission from Gimbel HV, Anderson Penno EE. *LASIK Complications: Prevention and Management.* Thorofare, NJ: SLACK Incorporated, 1999.)

LASIK After Cataract Surgery

This 74-year-old female presented to our clinic 14 years after cataract surgery OS and 1 month after cataract surgery OD. She remained myopic after surgery. Her UCVA OD was 20/70 with a manifest refraction of plano -2.25 x 116 corrected to 20/15 OD. The UCVA was 20/CF with a manifest refraction of -5.75 -2.25 x 92 corrected to 20/20 OS. She had no corneal pathology OU. She was in good medical health, took blood pressure medication, and had no drug allergies. We elected to perform LASIK OS only, as she might be able to tolerate spectacle correction OD after surgery.

On postoperative day 1, she had a UCVA of 20/50 $^{-3}$ which pinholed to 20/40 OS. At the 1-month follow-up examination, she had a UCVA of 20/50 $^{+2}$ with a manifest refraction of -1.00 -1.00 x 75 corrected to 20/25 $^{-2}$. There was a small nest of epithelial ingrowth, noted inferiorly. She is currently being followed for the epithelial ingrowth which will be removed if it shows progression.

This case illustrates that LASIK surgery can be safely performed following cataract surgery to correct anisometropia. It also illustrates that LASIK can be performed on patients of all ages—provided that they have healthy corneas. As the field of ophthalmology evolves and the demand for good UCVA increases, LASIK after cataract surgery will likely become more common.

PATIENT EXAMPLE 36

LASIK OS/PRK OD

This was a 39-year-old man in good health and with no medical problems. He requested to have his eyes done 1 month apart and decided on LASIK. Manifest refraction was -0.75 -1.75 x 172 OD and -1.75 -0.75 x 10 OS. BCVA was 20/20 OU. Manual keratometry was 41.37 @ 168 x 43.25 @ 78OD, 42.00 @ 178 x 43.37 @ 88 OS. LASIK was performed OS. It was noted that the epithelium was practically all denuded after the microkeratome pass. At the postoperative check, it was noted that there was a foreign body under the flap and a second foreign body under the contact lens that had been placed. The patient was taken back to the operating room, the contact lens was removed, and further irrigation was done under the flap in an unsuccessful attempt to remove interface debris. The flap was lifted and turned back, and the Paton spatula was used to brush away the interface debris. The flap was then replaced to the original position. The epithelium was brushed back into place using a dry Merocel sponge. Inspection now revealed a new foreign body. The flap was lifted and turned back again. A forceps was used to pick out a small filament of debris. The corneal flap was then moistened and replaced to the original position. Gentle irrigation under the flap was done and the fluid gently expressed. A contact lens was then replaced OS.

The patient was placed on topical antibiotic and steroid drops for the first week. At 5 days postoperative, the VASC was 20/50[-1], and manifest vision was 20/30[-2]. A corneal exam revealed trace epithelial irregularity, otherwise the flap was in good position. Four weeks postoperatively, VASC improved to 20/25[-3] with BCVA of 20/20[-2] with a manifest of plano -0.75 x 10. The slit lamp exam revealed trace diffuse haze with clearing of the interface haze. The patient and the surgeon elected to perform PRK on the right eye because of the probable unstable epithelium in this eye as well.

At 3 months postoperative PRK OD and 6 months postoperative LASIK OS, VASC OD was 20/15[-2] and VASC OS was 20/20[+2]. BCVA OD was 20/15 and 20/20 OS.

In this case, the complications encountered on the LASIK eye negated the benefits of rapid healing that are usually attributed to LASIK. Therefore, PRK was performed in the fellow eye with good results. This patient was in an excellent range for PRK.

(Reprinted with permission from Gimbel HV, Anderson Penno EE. *LASIK Complications: Prevention and Management.* Thorofare, NJ: SLACK Incorporated, 1999.)

PATIENT EXAMPLE 37

Pecan Injury 3 Months After LASIK

Three months after uncomplicated LASIK for -2.50 -0.75 @ 40 OD and -2.00 -0.50 @ 145 OS, this patient suffered a direct blow to the eye from a pecan falling from a tree. Her uncorrected vision prior to the injury was 20/20⁻ OU. She presented to the eye center approximately 48 hours after the injury with decreased acuity, upper and lower lid edema, and a flap that was folded over the nasal third. In addition, significant debris was imbedded on the surface as well as under the dislodged portion of the flap.

Due to the delay in presentation the bed had re-epithelialized and had to be debrided. The surface was debrided and the nasal flap was refloated into position. At 1 day postoperative, the patient had 1+ Descemet's folds, 2+ infection and 1+ cell, and flare UCVA was 20/100. The patient was maintained on topical steroid, topical NSAID and broad spectrum antibiotic. The patient was seen daily, and by the 1-week check, the uncorrected vision recovered to 20/20⁻³ and the eye was quiet. At the last exam 4 months postoperatively, the flap remained in good position with slight interface haze nasally and no sign of epithelial ingrowth.

This case shows the risk of flap dislocation with direct ocular trauma even 3 months postoperatively. It is important when presentation is delayed to carefully debride epithelium on the bed to avoid later epithelial ingrowth.

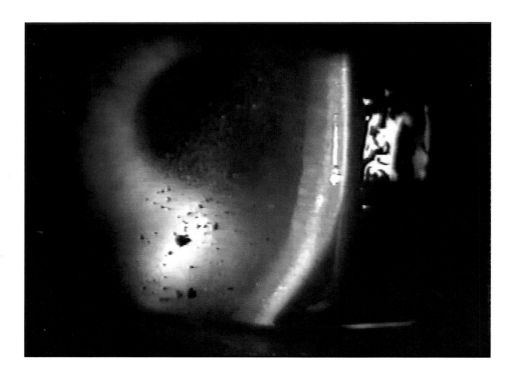

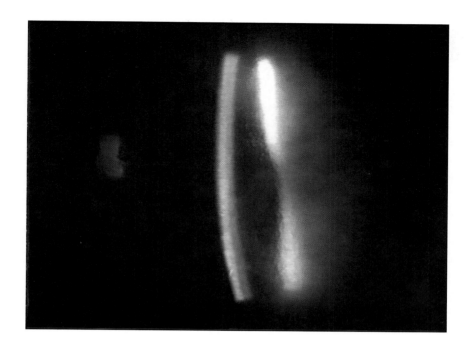

PATIENT EXAMPLE 38

Cable Injury 10 Months After LASIK

This 32-year-old independent contractor underwent uncomplicated LASIK OU for -2.75 -1.00 x 8 OD and -2.75 -1.5 x 159 OS. The assessment and postoperative exam was unremarkable with a UCVA of 20/20⁻¹ OD and 20/15⁻² OS at 3 months postoperatively. Approximately 11 months postoperatively, the patient was hit in the left eye with a cable at work. He presented to the clinic within a few hours of the injury stating that the eye was comfortable and central vision was clear; however, he noticed peripheral distortion. Uncorrected vision was 20/20⁺² with a temporal flap dislocation with microfolds and a widened gutter between 1:30 and 6:00 o'clock. The patient was taken to the operating suite where the temporal portion of the flap was refloated into position after clearing epithelial remnants from the edge of the bed. The patient maintained 20/20 UCVA.

This case demonstrates the risk of late flap dislocation with direct corneal trauma and emphasizes the need for safety glasses when working in high-risk environments. In this case there were only minimal indications by history of a dislodged flap. Therefore, all patients with a history of ocular trauma should be instructed to have an eye exam regardless of symptoms.

PATIENT EXAMPLE 39

Airbag Injury 34 Months After LASIK

At her initial refractive assessment, this 20-year-old had a manifest refraction of -9.00 -1.75 x 20 OD and -9.25 -2.00 x 150 OS with a BCVA of 20/20⁻² OU. LASIK was performed OU, and the patient did very well postoperatively Visual acuity at 6 months was 20/25⁺² OD and 20/25⁻¹ OS uncorrected. The refraction was plano -0.50 x 150 OD and +0.25 -0.50 x 50 OS with a BCVA of 20/20⁻² OU.

At 2 years and 10 months postoperative LASIK, the patient had a motor vehicle accident in which the air bag deployed and forced her knuckles into her orbit OD. She was treated for related trauma and a soft tissue infection of her face and presented to the center approximately 1 week after trauma. On examination, the UCVA was 20/20⁻² OD and 20/20⁻³ OS. Slit lamp exam revealed displacement and wrinkling of the flap superotemporally in the right eye. The original flap was made with the ACS, and the patient was taken to the operating room where the flap was turned back approximately 50%. The epithelium was carefully cleared at the edges of the flap and bed. The flap was then replaced and stretched to remove the microwrinkles. At 1 day postoperatively, UCVA was 20/20⁻³ and the patient noted improvement in the quality of vision. The slit lamp exam revealed trace microstriations and slight epithelial irregularity.

This case demonstrates that with significant direct trauma even many months to years after surgery, there is a risk for flap dislocation. In addition, this case also demonstrates that with appropriate treatment even 1 week after the flap dislocation, an excellent result can be obtained.

PATIENT EXAMPLE 40

Recutting With a Hansatome Over an Old Hyperopic ACS for the Treatment of Residual Hyperopia

This 45-year-old female underwent primary LASIK for hyperopic astigmatism OU. She was in good medical health, used only naprosin pills, and had no drug allergies. At that time, her flaps were made with an ACS microkeratome using a 160 µ depth plate. Her manifest refraction on assessment was +3.00 -1.00 x 155 corrected to 20/20 OD and +4.75 -1.50 x 07 corrected to 20/40 vision OS. She was amblyopic OS. Surgery OU was unremarkable.

Three months postoperatively, she remained undercorrected with a manifest refraction of +2.00 -0.75 x 165 corrected to 20/20 OD and +3.25 -1.00 x 173 corrected to 20/40. The flaps were lifted and an enhancement was performed OU.

She returned 1 year later and had a UCVA of 20/25[-1] with a cycloplegic refraction of +4.25 -1.00 x 147 corrected to 20/20[-1] OD, and a UCVA of 20/70 with a cycloplegic refraction of +4.75 -1.50 x 178 corrected to 20/40[-2] OS. Her previous ACS flap was too narrow to allow a 9.0 mm transition zone for hyperopic treatment, so a new flap was cut OU using the Hansatome.

The depth plate used on the first eye (OS) was 180 µ. After reflecting the flap, a thin loose sliver of stroma was noted on the undersurface of the cap. The planned ablation was performed. The sliver was wrinkled and directly in the visual axis. With difficulty, it was smoothed and the flap repositioned. The second eye (OD) was then cut using a 160 µ depth plate to try to avoid this same difficulty. After reflecting the flap there were two thin loose slivers of stroma on the bed, and both slivers were outside the visual axis. Again, the planned ablation was performed, and the slivers were much easier to smooth into position due to the support provided by the globe.

On postoperative day 1, she had a UCVA of 20/50 OD and 20/125 OS. She pinholed to 20/40 OD and 20/80[-2]. The flaps were in good position OU with no wrinkles or folds. There were mild SPK OU. Her UCVA improved to 20/25[-] OD with a manifest refraction of -0.25 -0.50 x 170 corrected to 20/25. UCVA OS was 20/60 with a manifest refraction of -0.50 -0.50 x 122 corrected to 20/50. At her 3-month visit, her UCVA OD was 20/25[+1] with a manifest refraction of +1.00 -0.50 x 175 corrected to 20/25[+1]. UCVA OS was 20/60[-2] with a manifest refraction of +1.75 - 0.25 x 15 corrected to 20/50.

It is always preferable to lift the flap instead of recutting if possible. Recutting the flap may lead to thin slivers that may be difficult to manage, similar to this case. We now only recommend recutting the flap for enhancement after 12 months following hyperopic LASIK in cases in which a small flap has been previously used. If recutting is necessary, we recommend recutting at the same depth as the original flap to avoid central slivers on the undersurface of the cap that might be quite difficult to manage. In cases in which an enhancement is performed within 12 months of the primary procedure, or if a 9.5 mm or 10.0 mm flap was used, and is well-centered, and the ablation was within the edges of the bed, we recommend relifting the flap (even after 24 to 36 months following the primary procedure).

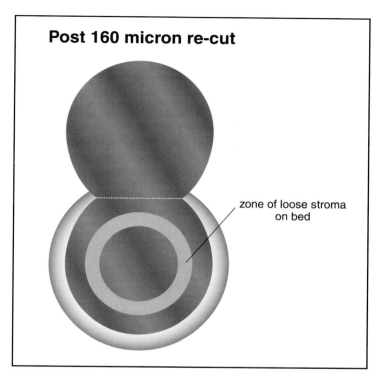

Post 160 micron re-cut

zone of loose stroma
on bed

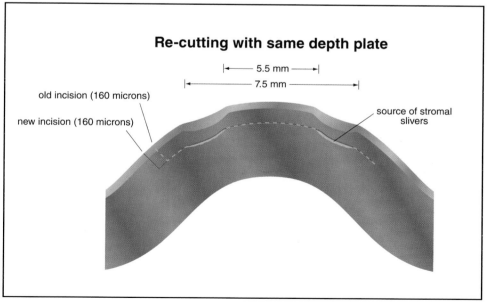

Re-cutting with same depth plate

|← 5.5 mm →|

|← 7.5 mm →|

old incision (160 microns)

new incision (160 microns)

source of stromal
slivers

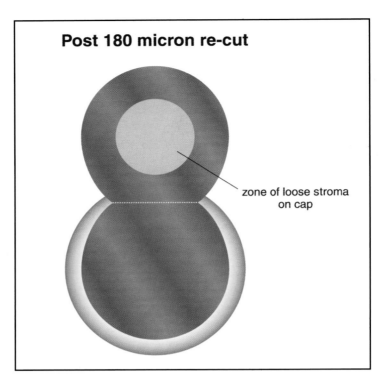

Post 180 micron re-cut

zone of loose stroma
on cap

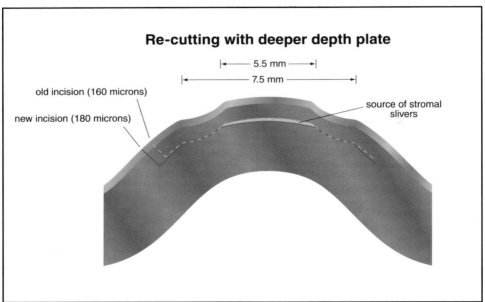

Re-cutting with deeper depth plate

|← 5.5 mm →|

|← 7.5 mm →|

old incision (160 microns)

new incision (180 microns)

source of stromal
slivers

PATIENT EXAMPLE 41

LASIK with Nystagmus

This 56-year-old male presented for LASIK for myopic astigmatism OU. He was in good health, took no medications, and no known drug allergies. He had a past ocular history of congenital rotary nystagmus and mild amblyopia OU. His manifest refraction on assessment was -3.50 -1.50 x 9 best-corrected to 20/20- 3 OD, and -4.75 -0.50 x 143 best-corrected to 20/20- 3 OS.

Intraoperatively, the patient's eye and head were fixated with a two-hand technique. one hand was placed on the forehead to stabilize the head, and a Gimbel-Thronton fixation ring was used with the other hand to overcome the nystagmus (care was taken when applying this pressure to not tort the eye). Excellent stability and centration were maintained throughout the procedure.

On postoperative day 1, his UCVA was 20/30- 1 pinholed to 20/20- 1 OD, and 20/30-1 pinholed to 20/20- 2 OS. Subjectively, the patient reported his vision was better than before surgery with his glasses.

This case demonstrates that LASIK can be performed safely and sucessfully under certain circumstances in nystagmus patients. The routine use of a fixation ring in all cases is recommended in order to transfer the skills required to use a fixation ring in nystagmus patients.

Index

.

BUILD Your Library

This book and many others on numerous different topics are available from SLACK Incorporated. For further information or a copy of our latest catalog, contact us at:

Professional Book Division
SLACK Incorporated
6900 Grove Road
Thorofare, NJ 08086 USA
Telephone: 1-856-848-1000
1-800-257-8290
Fax: 1-856-853-5991
E-mail: orders@slackinc.com
www.slackbooks.com

We accept most major credit cards and checks or money orders in US dollars drawn on a US bank. Most orders are shipped within 72 hours.

Contact us for information on recent releases, forthcoming titles, and bestsellers. If you have a comment about this title or see a need for a new book, direct your correspondence to the Editorial Director at the above address.

Thank you for your interest and we hope you found this work beneficial.